EBOLA

Andy Dennis and Anna Simon

# EBOLA

*behind the mask*

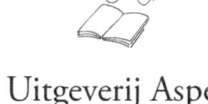

Uitgeverij Aspekt

EBOLA

© 2016 Uitgeverij ASPEKt
© Andy Dennis and Anna Simon

Amersfoortsestraat 27, 3769 AD Soesterberg, Nederland
info@uitgeverijaspekt.nl
http://www.uitgeverijaspekt.nl

Cover design and support throughout the production of this book: ARRIS www.arris.co.uk
Inside: Salihanur Akpinar

ISBN: 9789461539458
NUR: 870

All rights reserved. No reproduction copy or transmission of this publication may be made without written permission.

This book is dedicated to the people of Sierra Leone whose lives were touched by the tragedy of Ebola.

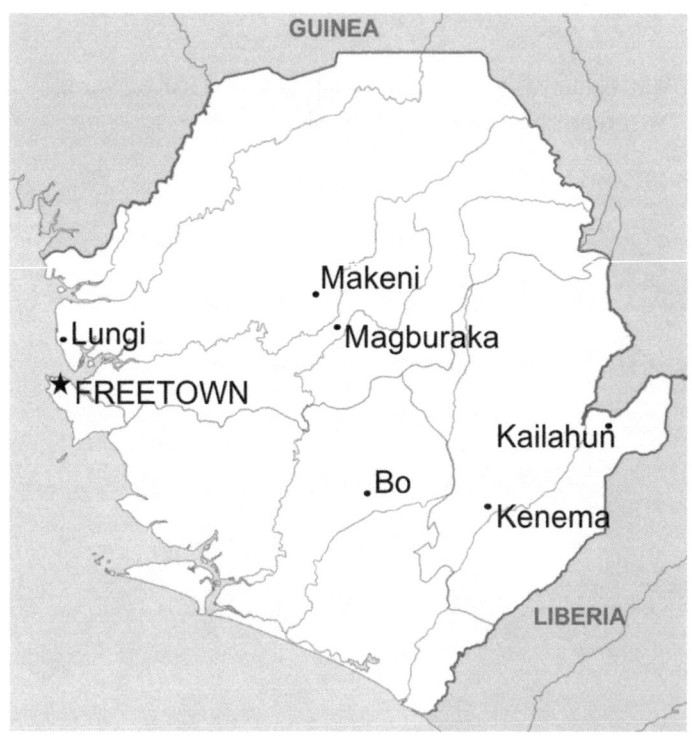

*Sierra Leone*

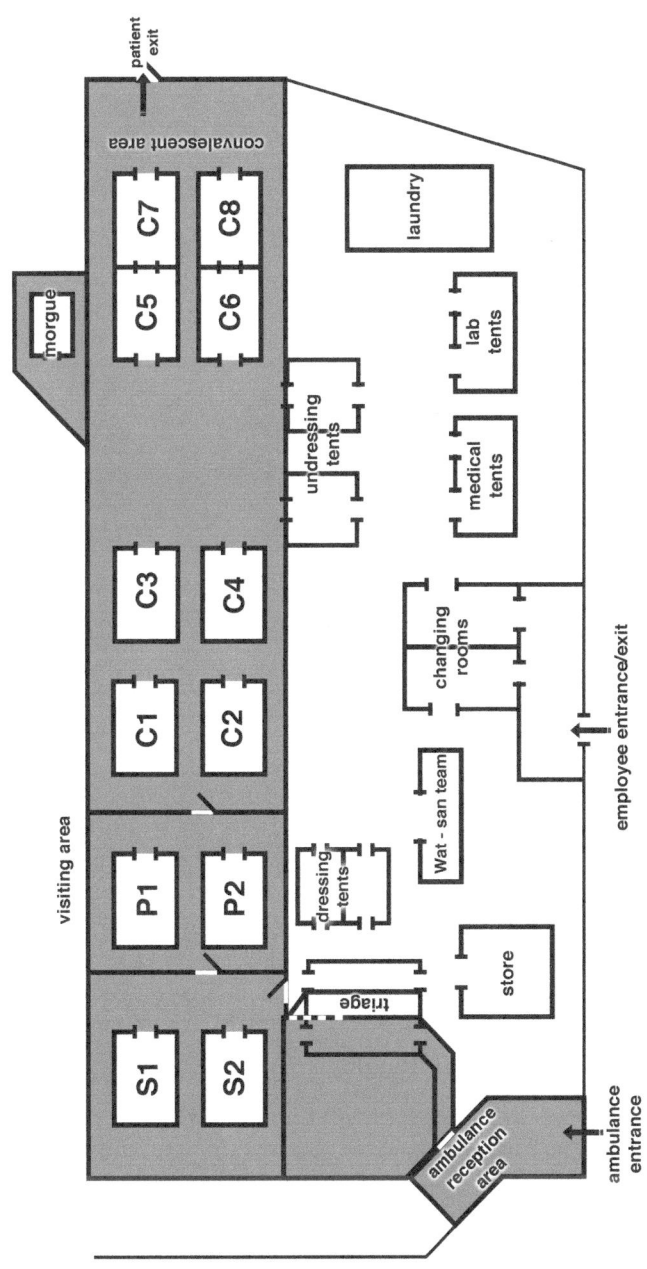

Simplified plan of the EMC in Kailahun. Shaded gray area is the High Risk zone.

# Foreword

The Ebola outbreak in West Africa was the worst public health emergency of modern times. But the world was slow to respond, and the consequences were dire.

Whilst much of the world recoiled in fear as images of the growing crisis were beamed across the globe, there was a small army of fighters preparing to head straight into the danger zone. They were doctors, nurses, psychologists, epidemiologists, laboratory staff and logisticians – to name just a few. They joined forces with the national medical staff, whose brave efforts were simply not enough for an outbreak that was already out of control. More than 500 West African health care workers died of Ebola in Sierra Leone, Liberia and Guinea.

I started covering the outbreak for BBC News towards the end of March 2014, when the medical charity Médecins Sans Frontières declared that an "unprecedented" Ebola epidemic was underway. By July I was reporting from West Africa's first Ebola treatment centre in the remote forested region of Guéckédou, South East Guinea where the outbreak began. I have never experienced such palpable fear as when I visited one particular community there. It hung thick in the air and was clear to see on so many people's faces. It's something that will stay with me for a very long time.

It's difficult to over-state the challenge those responding to this outbreak faced. As well as fear, there was a great deal of mistrust, suspicion and denial about Ebola, particularly in the early months of the outbreak. This was compounded by a lack of information about the virus and how it's spread. On that first trip to Guéckédou, I travelled with medics and communication teams into a village that had suffered a spate of mysterious deaths. They spent time explaining to residents what Ebola was and made it clear – with the help of a recent Ebola survivor – that the virus was not an automatic death sentence. Within an hour, people had started bringing out their sick relatives. There were many of them that day.

During my various deployments to some of the worst affected areas between 2014-2015, I reported from 9 different Ebola treatment centres. We always stayed in the low-risk zones, which were a safe distance away from sick patients. We'd watch medical staff carefully step into their personal protective gear, and disappear into the high-risk areas, where many people were dying.

I interviewed dozens of health workers to find out what life was really like for them behind that mask. How did it feel seeing so many patients who were extremely unwell and knowing that the help you could give them was limited to supportive treatments?
There wasn't – and still isn't – a proven cure for Ebola.

At the time those medics I spoke to were stoical and practical about the job at hand. Their general response was: "we just have to get on with it and do the best we can for patients".

It must have been difficult for them to try and process these extraordinary experiences whilst they themselves were still so close to the crisis.

In Ebola: *Behind the Mask*, Andy Dennis and Anna Simon take you right inside those hot claustrophobic Ebola treatment tents. Through their vivid accounts, you sit with them at the bedsides of patients they cared for.

Among them; 2-year-old little Kadiatu who was all alone as she fought for her life, Alimany the once strapping young Chelsea supporter, and 9-year-old Osman and his father – battling Ebola alongside each other. We see each of them through Andy and Anna's eyes, not just as numbers in a list of grim statistics, but as people who had once loved, laughed and lived.

The medics who fought Ebola are modern day heroes. In particular, as Anna and Andy point out, the hundreds of West African staff who fought the hardest, and paid the heaviest price.

The stories Anna and Andy share about their experiences and the people they cared for expose why the world must never allow a tragedy like this unfold again. It chronicles unimaginable fear, loss and chaos, but also shows great humanity, bravery and love.

Tulip Mazumdar, Global Health Correspondent, BBC News

# Introduction

*Andy Dennis:*
*Alimany the midfielder died last night. A young man in the prime of his life robbed of his future... I take a walk over to a secluded corner... Here I stand and stare into space. My thoughts and emotions swirl and, as often occurs here, I find myself with a deep sense of sorrow.*

*I have to collect myself quickly as this place is about the living and I have blood samples to collect.*

This book tells of the personal experiences of Andy Dennis and Anna Simon in Sierra Leone working for Doctors Without Borders / Médecins Sans Frontières (MSF) during the Ebola outbreak in 2014. It is based on the personal journals that they kept; and their combined different backgrounds and personalities gives a diverse insight into events as they unfolded.

In the four to five weeks that they worked in Kailahun, a remote province of Sierra Leone, they cared for more than 150 Ebola patients, assisting them in their recovery or ensuring a dignified death. They lived and worked in Kailahun but are not experts on West Africa in general or Sierra Leone in particular nor do they intend to give a full overview of the development of the outbreak, the response of the Western world or the efforts of the various other aid organisations.

Twenty-five patients that they cared for in their work are highlighted to give the story a personal touch. After all, they are the human faces engulfed by this crisis. The names of the people involved were changed, for privacy reasons, but their stories are true.

*MSF and their call for doctors and nurses*
MSF is an international medical emergency aid organisation whose goal is to provide medical care in areas where people have very limited or no access to it. It is active in more than 60 countries, often in areas that are hardly reached by other aid organisations: war zones, displaced populations, natural disasters or outbreaks of infectious diseases, or a combination of those. The central principle of MSF is that it remains neutral and impartial, and will help people irrespective of their background, religion or political preferences. This independence is strongly guarded. Doctors, nurses and other personnel are usually sent on missions of 9 to 12 months. Exceptions to this include emergency situations such as an Ebola outbreak or a natural disaster. In those cases, MSF can send the first people and supplies within 48 hours, to start up a rescue effort.

In the past, MSF has gained expertise in the response to the usual small, contained, Ebola outbreaks, for example in Congo. It has the protocols ready and a list of experienced doctors and nurses who can be sent to such an epidemic within a short period of time. MSF responded rapidly to this outbreak once the disease was recognised but this time the epidemic grew rapidly to unprecedented size. MSF sent more and more people, built more Ebola management centres and was active in keeping the world informed about the huge scale of the problem, to raise awareness that more help was needed.

By the end of September 2014, MSF needed so many new aid workers that it started to recruit doctors and nurses from outside the organisation. That is not a first: for example, specialised surgeons are sent to established MSF missions in war zones, to perform surgery for two to three weeks.

However, the scale of the call for help in The Netherlands, and especially the publicity surrounding it, was remarkable. Everything about Ebola became big news. The Dutch Minister of Health sent a letter to all Dutch hospitals in support of MSF, asking hospital directors to enable their employees to go if they wanted to. The requirements for doctors were straightforward: at least two years' experience as a medical doctor, experience in supervising others, a good knowledge of the English language and the ability to work in an international group of people. Desirable qualities were knowledge of contagious diseases, having worked for an aid organisation before or experience with medical care in a tropical country.

*Andy Dennis*

Andy has been a qualified nurse since 1995, prior to which he was a Royal Air Force Medical Assistant. He left the RAF in 1991 after the first Gulf War having decided that if he were to be in conflict situations again it was going to be in a humanitarian rather than a military role.

He has spent most of his career as a nurse working in the British National Health Service, predominantly in critical care areas such as Emergency Departments and Intensive Care. In 2004 he watched the global response to the Asian Tsunami. He stood in awe of one particular organisation and by June 2005 he was working as a nurse with Doctors Without Borders. His first mission was in Northern Uganda caring for people displaced by conflict with the Lord's Resistance Army (LRA).

Andy has subsequently worked in South Sudan on two occasions. In 2008 he was in Yambio near the border with the

Democratic Republic of Congo where he was helping to set up Primary Health Care clinics in two remote areas. This mission was also affected by violence perpetrated by the LRA; indeed, two people were killed in an attack on one of the clinics in late 2008. In 2013 Andy ran the nutrition programme at Leer Hospital in the North of the country. This Hospital had stood for 25 years, before its destruction a matter of weeks after he left in January 2014. He now works in the Endoscopy Department at Harrogate District Hospital, UK.

*Anna Simon*
Anna is a consultant in internal medicine and infectious diseases. She works in the Radboud University Medical Centre in Nijmegen, The Netherlands, combining patient care with scientific research and teaching. Her specialist subject is very rare hereditary disorders in the immunological field. She lived and worked in the USA for two years doing post-doctoral research in 2006-2007 but she had never worked in patient care outside of The Netherlands. At the beginning of October 2014, Anna responded to MSF's call for doctors and nurses to volunteer to work in the Ebola epidemic, which made headlines in The Netherlands, and she was accepted.

# Sunday, November 30, 2014

**Anna**

On the stretcher is a man of about 30 years of age. He groans a little but does not respond when Amara, the community health officer (CHO), asks him his name. He arrived yesterday, at the end of the afternoon, in an ambulance from Freetown (around seven hours drive from Kailahun). Of the five other patients in the ambulance, one had died en route. None of the other patients knew his identity.

I squat down next to the bed, carefully avoiding the pool of vomit on the floor, and not too close to his face in case he vomits again. The man's face is sunken and there is dried blood on his lips. I take hold of his arm. Through two layers of gloves I can hardly feel the weak, rapid pulse. The patient turns his face towards me when I touch him but he does not make eye contact. Amara has put a thermometer in the man's armpit: 39.2 degrees Celsius. I put my hand on his stomach. The slightest touch is obviously very painful. In his diaper I see diarrhoea mixed with blood. Officially, we do not know whether the patient has Ebola or not – the test result will come back in the afternoon – but I do not doubt that the test will be positive.

Slowly, I get to my feet. Amara and I exchange a knowing look from behind our safety goggles. I shake my head. "It's too late for him, we will just have to give him more pain medication and keep him comfortable." Amara nods, and with the help of Sheku, the nurse, he sets to work to clean the man. Sahr, the sprayer, stands at the ready with his CHLORINE spray to decontaminate my gloved hands. After that, he cleans the vomit from the floor.

Meanwhile I leave the tent and walk to the fence that separates the 'High Risk' and 'Low Risk' areas. I call for a medic. Quickly, a nurse walks up to me from within the Low Risk area. I ask her to prepare a syringe with morphine for pain and also something to help his nausea. Back inside the tent, I assist Sheku to prop the man up in bed, to see whether he can manage a drink. Amara is already helping the woman in the next bed. A couple of minutes later, a call from the fence: the medication has arrived.

Calmly, I get up and I walk slowly to the fence to collect the syringes. In full 'personal protective equipment' (PPE) inside the High Risk zone the last thing you want to do is trip and fall, or hit your head against the wooden beams, which were not built with tall Dutch women in mind. The temperature inside the PPE rises quickly, especially under a bright sun, even though it is not yet ten o'clock in the morning. I can feel the sweat trickling down my back, my socks squelch inside my boots. We were trained never to hurry inside the High Risk zone of the Ebola Management Centre, whatever the situation.

Back at the bedside, I give the man two injections in his upper leg, and immediately place the needles in a special safe container. That is all the time we have for the man at present. Amara, Sheku and I have been at work in our PPE in the High Risk zone for more than ten minutes already. We are tasked to see and help out

14 more ill patients before the hour is over and our time will be up.

Working inside the High Risk zone, you focus one hundred per cent on your job. Only when I return to the Low Risk zone and am more comfortably dressed in fresh surgical scrubs do I have time to sit down and rest. That is when my thoughts can wander a little. Sitting down with a bottle of water in the shade of the medical tent I think back to the last Sunday I spent at home, before leaving for Sierra Leone. That was only three weeks ago.

# Sunday, November 9

**Anna**

I'm in my study, gazing across the roofs of Nijmegen. I have been working since the early morning. Now my suitcase for Sierra Leone is packed, I can use the rest of the day for my 'work' to-do list – the list of things that need to be done to leave my 'normal' work in order. Writing letters about patients, cancelling appointments for the next two months, working on research projects, delegating teaching duties and cleaning up the dreaded email inbox.

Next week at this time, I will be somewhere in Sierra Leone. I think back to how I got to this position. As infectious disease specialists, my colleagues and I had been aware for some time of the growing Ebola epidemic in West Africa. Since the beginning of the summer, preparations have been made in our university hospital, the Radboud University Medical Center in Nijmegen, to enable us to look safely after a patient with suspected Ebola. My colleague Chantal coordinates this effort and, since we share a room at the hospital, I have followed developments as they happened. At the end of August, we started the actual training in the use of protective equipment.

On Monday September 22, after months of polishing up the details, the hospital Ebola protocols were completed and approved. As if it was meant to be, that same day our first suspected Ebola patient arrived and the protocols were put into action immediately. I was part of the team of doctors and nurses ready to care for him in strict isolation in a blocked off wing of our Infectious Diseases ward. But my turn only started on Tuesday evening, after finishing my outpatient clinic for the afternoon. The patient was not very ill. The results of his first test for Ebola had already come back negative, and he had tested positive for malaria. There was no reason for me to enter the patient's room, he was doing fine, so I did not need to put on the PPE (personal protective equipment) this time. During my shift, the long-awaited results from his second Ebola test came in: the patient did not have Ebola. All that was left for me to do was to give him and the nursing team the good news and end the strict isolation protocol.

*Ebola and this epidemic*
In brief, what is Ebola? The Ebola virus causes a disease characterised by fever, diarrhoea, vomiting, muscle ache and other symptoms. Just like any other viral disease, the combination and severity of the symptoms can vary drastically from person to person. As in influenza, for example, which causes one person to take to his bed with a high fever for a week, while the next gets by with three days of slightly raised temperature, muscle aches and general malaise.

Some patients with Ebola suffer from a few days of fever, diarrhoea, vomiting and muscle aches, before they start to recover spontaneously. Others have a more severe disease course; they get progressively ill, weak and bedridden. They suffer from increasing pain in their muscles, joints and stomach, and deteriorate rapidly. In the end stage of Ebola, they can experience internal bleeding, for example in the stomach, gut or lungs. Sometimes, they suffer from annoying, unstoppable hiccups – we don't know exactly why that happens. These are clear signs of the deadly form of the disease. Some people die quite suddenly.

It is hard to predict who will do well and who will not. The elderly, very young children and pregnant women have a high risk of death. But young twenty-somethings, who were completely healthy before, can also die within a few days.

Perhaps some people can be contaminated with the Ebola virus while they show little or no symptoms. That happens in almost all infectious diseases, from the common cold to the Q-fever bacterium. We suspect so, but no evidence for this has been collected as yet.

In the past 40 years, since the first description of the Ebola virus, there has been only limited research into the characteristics of the virus or the disease it causes in humans. This has to do with the fact that it only strikes in remote, poor regions of Africa. Every year, until last year. small Ebola epidemics occurred, particularly in Eastern and Middle Africa. Of course, it is not easy to conduct scientific research on this deadly virus.

This outbreak started in December 2013 in Guinea. It took a couple of months before it was clear that the Ebola virus caused it. This disease had never before occurred in West Africa. By the summer of 2014 the epidemic was spreading rampantly, especially in the border area of the three countries of Guinea, Sierra Leone and Liberia. In September and October 2014 when a number of cases ended up in the Western world and the epidemic became more and more out of control in West Africa, Ebola finally gained prominence in the world news.

Through Chantal, I learned early on that MSF was urgently looking for experienced doctors and nurses who were willing to work in one of their Ebola Management Centres (EMCs) in West Africa. I thought they would have trouble finding anyone. Who has "experience" in Ebola? But when I heard that two nurses from our department were planning to apply, and MSF's appeal reached the national news, I started to consider it more seriously myself. I don't have a partner or children and no dependent relatives, which makes the decision easier.

Finally, after a couple of weeks of thinking about it, mostly in secret, on Friday October 10 I decided to follow my heart. The first step was telling my colleagues at our weekly meeting. "I hope you won't burst out laughing, but I have been thinking about it, and I want to get in touch with MSF, and put in an application to work as a doctor in an Ebola centre – if you agree to it."

I really thought they would have laughed: Anna, going to Africa? I have never even been in a tropical country and my daily work is far removed from tropical diseases. But they responded positively.

That same evening, right after work, I sent a carefully formulated application email to MSF. If I'm totally honest, at this point I was still secretly hoping that they would reject me: that would have meant I had done my best and I didn't really have to go and could stay here in my comfort zone.

But my application to MSF was received favourably. I was invited to an interview, had a psychological assessment and was accepted within three weeks of that first contact. All that remained unclear was the timing. The MSF coordinator promised to let me know the options by the first week of November.

On Tuesday afternoon November 4 I was busy with my outpatient clinic but between patients I couldn't stop myself from checking my email. A message from MSF. Two options: either leaving in March or leaving on November 15 because someone has had to withdraw at the last minute. Leaving in ten days time! Which would mean starting the training in eight days time! My heart pounded in my chest as I quickly closed the email. Three more patients to go, no time to think about it now, these patients deserve my full attention.

Three quarters of an hour later, when I finished my clinic, I started to realise what this meant. If I said yes, I would be boarding a plane to Sierra Leone in 10 days time! By this time, I really wanted to go. I thought I should be able to get everything organised and I would actually leave less work behind for my colleagues now than if I left in March. My superiors were also overwhelmed by the short notice but their support was clear from the start. On Wednesday November 5, I received the go ahead from my department, and I let the MSF coordinator know that I was willing and able to fill in the November 15 departure spot.

This left me with five working days and two weekend days before the start of the training followed directly by the mission to Sierra Leone. During this week, emails from several departments of MSF kept dropping in – containing briefing documents about the country, the mission, the insurance policies, forms that needed to be filled about my health, my contact information, a visa application, lists of necessary vaccination, information about the training in Amsterdam and flight details.

Meanwhile, my regular work continues as if nothing had happened. This forces me to think about something other than MSF and Ebola, which is a good thing. The to-do list gets longer and longer, and I work long evenings to get everything sorted.

I'm fully supported by my hospital: they grant me paid leave. All my colleagues and others in the hospital respond in a positive way. "You actually look more relaxed than you did last week," a colleague told me. He was right. I felt better now that the time of waiting and insecurity was over.

Yesterday I went into town with my shopping list. I've had all kinds of advice from my colleagues with experience of working in the tropics and from MSF, about what to take. Today, my suitcase is practically ready. This time next week I will be in Freetown.

# Monday, November 10

**Anna**
A regular working day – but not really. In between seeing some unsuspecting patients in the outpatient clinic, I get seven vaccinations, including yellow fever, tetanus, and hepatitis A, and make copies of documents I need for the journey.

Several colleagues ask, "Why are you going?" I had that same question from some friends last weekend. For me it is more relevant to ask, "Why wouldn't I?" Help is desperately needed, even more than money, and I may be qualified to provide that help. I also look at it in reverse: what if there were some deadly illness going around in my own country and for some reason the healthcare system had broken down and couldn't handle it – I would wish that people from other 'safe' countries would be prepared to risk their lives to come and help us. So, I should be willing to do the same, as I may be able to in this case.

Around noon, I have to deliver a lecture for second year medical students. They are in the middle of a teaching course on Infectious Diseases. One of the lecture slots in the series is always left open, to be filled in last minute with a topical subject. This year, Ebola is an obvious choice. The large lecture hall is filled with between 300 and 400 young students.

Chantal starts off with a good presentation on the medical background of Ebola, about the epidemic and the organisation of the care of potential patients in The Netherlands. The students in the audience listen attentively. But afterwards, the only question comes from a female student in one of the first rows: "Which part of this do we actually have to know for the exam?"

Chantal and I exchange exasperated glances, but we control ourselves: we tell her to check that with the course coordinator. We suspect that there are a lot of students in the hall who are more mature and who are ashamed of their colleague's attitude.

Then it's my turn. I have not had time to prepare slides, it will be an off-the-cuff story. When I start by telling them that this Saturday I will be stepping on a plane to Sierra Leone to work for MSF, you can hear a pin drop in the lecture hall. I tell them what my work will be in an Ebola Management Centre and explain to them how such a centre works, using a picture from the MSF website. I talk to them about why I have chosen to apply for this, despite the risks.

Afterwards, I invite the students to ask questions. To break the tension in the room, I can't resist telling them that I think that this will not be part of the exam. This causes some sniggering. A number of serious, interested questions follow. Whether I'm scared that I will get Ebola myself. What my family thinks of my decision. At the end, unexpectedly the students give me resounding applause. A nice gesture from them, which touches me. That afternoon, a group of the students send me an email, to thank me for making them think and to wish me a successful and safe mission.

At the end of a long day, I'm tired. There is so much to get ready in such a short time, for the trip, for my personal affairs at home, for the work I leave behind – it drains my energy. Due to my fatigue I am somewhat bad tempered on the phone this evening with my parents, my brother Huib and my sister-in-law Mireille, but I know they understand me.

Every drawback has an advantage: the hectic but short time for preparation is extremely intense, but will also pass very quickly.

# Tuesday, November 11

**Andy**

It is ten o'clock in the evening in the Meininger Hotel in Amsterdam. I am going to bed in a few minutes, as tomorrow is a big day. I will be starting my "Ebola training" prior to heading to Sierra Leone on Saturday. I have spent much of the evening mulling over the events of the last few weeks and months.

In mid 2014 the world finally woke up to the Ebola outbreak in West Africa. I was losing sleep and finding myself unable to concentrate. How could I live with this situation as a distant voyeur when I have skills and knowledge that could help?

I had just started a new job at the Harrogate District Hospital's Endoscopy Department in August 2014. By the end of September I was in my boss's office after asking if she was free for a chat. "Lorraine, I have something I need to ask you" I began, before telling her the story of my sleepless nights and how I had a nagging sense of unease and frustration. "I am really suffering watching all of the news reports about Ebola and not being involved in the response. I have decided to just come out with it and ask you if there is any way I can have time off work for a mission." I explained that it would be a one-month mission but there would likely be a period of monitoring afterwards to ensure I am disease free. In my heart I hoped that Lorraine would say yes but I was acutely aware that she has responsibilities that may make it impossible for her to allow me to go. She listened intensely as I explained my request and then offered an immediate "yes." She followed this with a very moving explanation of why she believed this was an important thing for her to support both as a person and as a manager in our hospital.

I left the office feeling both elated and nervous. I was one step closer to my next mission. Later I called MSF to let them know that I had approval from work and asked that they actively look at matching me to a mission in West Africa.

The rapid turnover of staff in the missions is a nightmare to manage for the human resources team in the MSF offices. Due to the intensity of the work and the inherent risk of Ebola, missions for expat medical personnel who work inside the Ebola Management Centre (EMC) are limited to four or five weeks duration instead of the usual six months. The number of people required to staff the projects adequately is therefore immense. Finally and by email on October 20, 2014 I was offered a four-week mission in Kailahun, Eastern Sierra Leone.

Harrogate District Hospital is a close-knit community and I know many people who work there. Each day I was asked questions by people who had heard on the grapevine that I was going to work in the Ebola outbreak and wanted to express concern. "How long?" "Where?" "Will you be safe?" "What happens when you return?" Right up until I leave for Holland I am finding out information about the mission. The question about what happens at the end of my time in Sierra Leone will no doubt be answered in the next few weeks. There are many ambiguities about the 21-day monitoring period and its implications for coming back to work post mission. All will become clear, I am sure.

So here I lay in the Meininger Hotel, one and a half months down the line contemplating the coming weeks. I have been saying farewell to people for the last three weeks and today at Leeds Bradford Airport I said goodbye to my Mum and Dad and Tracey, my long-suffering girlfriend. I know that this is a lot to put them through, so many people are dying in this outbreak and the reports are all over the TV. There is little escape from the tragedy that is Ebola.

I try to clear my mind, I relax on my comfortable bed and turn off the light.

# Wednesday, November 12
# – Ebola training from MSF in Amsterdam

**Andy**

The night is rather unsettled, the change of environment, the saying goodbye, the anticipation of today, missing Tracey. It all adds up to disturbed sleep. I leave the room and go down for breakfast in the morning about quarter past seven with the plan to be out of the hotel by about half past seven. I soon identify other MSF people, which is both reassuring and interesting, there must be an MSF look! More likely it is the mixed group of people dressed in many different ways and the varieties of accents that make me suspect I have found my new colleagues. We leave the hotel as a group and head towards the bus station on our way to the MSF Ebola Training Centre.

An unexpected surprise is that one of the participants is a psychologist that visited the hospital in Leer South Sudan when I was there in 2013. Also Jeff, my former boss from South Sudan, is on the bus. It is very nice to see them as it is always a little strange meeting a whole new bunch of people and a familiar face just takes the edge off the nerves. Jeff and I have a quick catch up before getting to the Ebola Training Centre.

Inside the Ebola Training Centre, a fully set up treatment area is ready for us with High and Low Risk areas, manikin patients, chlorine points for hand washing and decontamination, dressing and undressing stations and everything else we need for our training.

The day is taken up with lectures and practical sessions in the simulation area. Lectures cover the Ebola epidemic, the management of the disease, the risks and how we can protect ourselves and how an EMC (Ebola Management Centre) works. In the afternoon, there's a practical exercise in the simulated EMC, to practise dressing and undressing in the personal protective equipment (PPE). One very important point that is emphasised is the need to respect and appreciate the National Staff. The Sierra Leonean staff have been working in the EMC in Kailahun since June and have been caring for and burying their colleagues, family and friends since then. The last thing they need is new expats going there every four to five weeks with totally new ways to do everything.

The other trainees seem like a nice group of people and we are slowly getting to know one another. Most of them are heading to Kailahun. There are of course one or two personalities that seem rather domineering and opinionated but I guess that's pretty normal.

We train until about six o'clock then eat pizza and enjoy a beer back at the hotel bar, chat and get to know each other in a social setting.

> *How contagious is Ebola actually?*
> Not very much. Especially compared to other viruses, for example the regular influenza virus. The Ebola virus cannot be spread through the air. It is destroyed by exposure to soap and water, or to water with added chlorine. Even UV-light from the sun is enough to kill the virus. And it is not able to pass through intact skin.

To get ill from the virus, you have to be in direct contact with body fluids from someone who is ill from Ebola. Diarrhoea, vomit, blood, sweat, tears, urine – every kind of body fluid. Next, the virus has to enter your system through either a breach of your skin, or through your mucosa such as eyes or mouth when you subconsciously touch your face and rub your eyes or touch your lips. If you get contaminated blood on your hand but directly clean it with water and soap without touching your face, nothing will happen providing, of course, that you do not have any cuts on your hand.

There are many safety measures to prevent contamination. The most effective measure is frequent hand washing, with water and soap, alcohol hand gel or chlorine water. This sounds easy, but it can be harder than you think in a country where running water is a luxury. Another safety measure is the instruction to keep a distance of 2 metres from an Ebola patient, and to avoid touching him. That distance is enough to keep you out of range of any vomit or coughing; the bigger drops of vomit that could potentially contain virus particles will fall in a range of about 1 metre.

In the EMC, there is an area called the High Risk zone where suspected and confirmed Ebola patients are cared for. Here, more strict safety protocols are in place. Everyone will have seen it on TV or on the internet. Anyone entering the High Risk zone dresses up in personal protective equipment (PPE). This covers the entire body and consists of an overall, an apron, a facemask, a hood to cover your head, double layers of gloves and finally big safety goggles. Not an inch of skin remains uncovered. Of course, you cannot maintain the safe distance from patients when caring for them. Patients need to be washed, vomit and diarrhoea needs to be cleaned up and patients have to be tended to after their death. All circumstances that will put you in close contact with the virus. Dressed in PPE the outside of your protective covering will become contaminated with virus. In between each patient-related action, you wash your double gloved hands in chlorine water. This also offers protection for the patients: even in the part of the EMC where every patient already suffers from Ebola, you do not want to spread regular bacteria from one to the other.

You never enter the High Risk zone on your own, but are always accompanied by at least one buddy. You keep an eye on each other: no tears in the gloves? Have the goggles shifted, to expose a bit of skin? Are you OK in the heat? You must leave before it is too late: As soon as you discover a breach of your PPE or you are exhausted or at the end of the maximum one hour allowed in High Risk.

Finally one of the most important parts of the safety protocol: the undressing. You know that there is likely to be Ebola virus on the outside of your PPE, so you want to take care not to be exposed to that during undressing. There's always a specially dedicated person to help you through the process step by step even if you've done it many times before. A careful undressing procedure will take about ten minutes.

In day to day life, you would not easily get contaminated by an Ebola patient in the Western world, where everyone has their own toothbrush, and their own knife and fork at dinner. Where a lot of people have never seen a real dead person, close up. Where every house has running water, and everyone can easily wash his or her hands. The few Ebola patients that have ended up in the West have never spread the disease to their house members or neighbours. The only contaminations outside Africa have been of nurses who cared for a patient when they were already ill in the hospital, and the right safety protocols were not in place.

# Thursday, November 13 – Second day of training

**Andy**

Around ten in the evening on Wednesday I say goodnight to Tracey over Skype and switch the light off hoping for a good night's sleep. However I lie awake with the day cascading through my mind. In the end I drift off sometime after midnight.

I wake suddenly at half past three. I had just been shown a mouth swab that had turned green indicating that I was positive for Ebola! It was a stupid dream but entirely understandable after the day that we had had. I lie back onto the pillow, smile to myself and contemplate what complex beings we really are.

We start at nine at the training centre today. The lectures cover medical case management, case finding and contact tracing. The case management lecture makes it very clear that we will have to adjust our expectations quite considerably when it comes to clinical interventions. There will be no complex equipment for monitoring patients and limited laboratory tests available. In the West, we are heavily dependent on these and there is a degree of anxiety from some of the trainees when they hear that they will not be available in Sierra Leone. This is, in fact, standard for MSF missions in my experience. Practitioners have to rely on their basic medical training and adapt to each situation.

After lunch we begin a sweat inducing practical session using our Italian logistics man Alessandro as a patient. Alessandro has a fine sense of humour, which I test with abusive comments and mockery: I can tell that we are going to get on well from the outset! I am sad that he is not going to be coming to Kailahun with me as his project is based in Bo, about four hours west of Kailahun. We spend the one hour maximum time we are allowed in the simulated High Risk area learning how to unload him from the ambulance, simulate taking some blood and finally how to undress from the PPE. By the time we remove the PPE we are soaked in sweat. It's November in Holland!

As the course progresses I feel an increasing sense of confidence both in MSF and in the other trainees. We talk about our feelings quite openly and how we are both nervous and keen to begin our work in the outbreak.

**Anna**

Two days of training about MSF and Ebola, and meeting my new colleagues. Besides myself, only two of the group have not worked with MSF previously. One of them is going to Sierra Leone to work for another organisation (MSF trains numerous people from other organisations), the other was recruited just like me. The other people are all experienced MSF-ers, swapping stories of previous missions, adventures in faraway countries and common acquaintances, and using MSF jargon with plenty of abbreviations. It is all very different from my ultra-academic background but they are a welcoming group. I'm very glad to know that I will be making the journey to

Sierra Leone with them, and will be working in the same EMC as some.

In the evening, I catch a bus to the village of Santpoort-Noord to the west of Amsterdam, to spend a night with my brother Huib and his wife Mireille. I have a good time at the dinner table with their three children. My nephews Wisse (seven years old) and Floris (six years old) know all about their aunt Anna travelling to Africa to help people ill with Ebola (two-year-old Emma is too young). They give me beautiful drawings to hang in my room while over there. Wisse warns me not to swim in water near a hippopotamus, because he has just learned from famous national children's TV biologist Freek that the hippo is the strongest animal in Africa and kills a lot of people every year.

# Friday, November 14 – Briefings

**Anna**

A day filled with briefings at the MSF Amsterdam head office, tightly planned. Individually meeting a psychologist, about my psychological well-being, a medical doctor, about my physical health now and later, someone from human resources about the contract, the Sierra Leone visa and a special MSF ID card. Group meetings about communications with the press and publicity and about the specific situation in the EMCs in Bo and Kailahun. I'm impressed by the smoothly run operation. This is a very big mission and all medics who go to work inside an EMC will stay for a maximum period of five weeks. Therefore people are being sent out and returning every week, to ensure an overlap. We also receive the beautiful white MSF T-shirts today. The atmosphere is good. These are ideal circumstances for quick and strong team building.

At half past five the day of briefings is over. I catch a train to Nijmegen to spend a final night in my own bed. My parents visit me to say goodbye. That isn't easy, but I feel strengthened by their support. I remember the way I broke the news to them that I had applied to MSF for this mission. My parents are both doctors, so in a way it is easier for them to understand my drive and accept the risks involved, but my mother is a worrier by nature so I felt bad about causing her extra anxiety. Even though she is very anxious, she is great about it – she would never stop me doing something because of her worries. For good luck, she has started a knitting project: together, we've picked out a pattern for a cardigan, which she will start as soon as I have left, and which will have to be finished before my return to ensure I come back safely. We plan to Facetime or Skype a lot; there should be Wi-Fi in the hotel in Kailahun, so that should be OK.

I also start on the malaria prophylaxis this evening. I'll buy a few last small things Saturday morning, and then everything is ready.

**Andy**
In the evening I take a tram to the centre of Amsterdam to do some last minute shopping. The training sessions made it clear that I needed to review my deodorant supply, I also buy some more socks and foot powder to treat fungal infections. Not a particularly attractive subject but from the training I can see that it is a potential complication of the work. As I walk in the city centre I think to myself how normal everything looks. I am mulling over the impending few weeks as I walk into Dam Square. I look up at the Royal Palace in all its splendour and try to imagine the Ebola Management Centre in Kailahun. As I cross the Square I see Death standing before me. The Grim Reaper stands tall and menacing, scythe in bony hand ready to lead me to the next world. I hold this image for a beat and then smile as a tourist stands next to the guy in the suit to have her photo taken. I won't be heading to my eternal resting place tonight.

I leave the centre and walk back as it starts to rain. I bump into Alessandro at the hotel and we head over the road to a pub. For the next three hours or so we drink too much beer and chat about past MSF experiences and the upcoming mission. It is about midnight when we return to the hotel.

# Saturday, November 15 – travelling to Freetown

**Andy**

Bloody Italian keeping me up till midnight drinking Belgian beer! I feel decidedly hung over this morning, not the best preparation for a near 24-hour journey.

We leave the hotel about two in the afternoon. I have a sense of foreboding on the way to the airport. I have suffered with a fear of flying since I was in an incident in a Puma helicopter in the First Gulf War when I was an RAF medical assistant. Sometime in February 1991 I was in the back of a Puma helicopter, having just dropped a patient off at a field hospital and returning to base in King Khaleds Military City (Saudi Arabia). About 15 minutes out of the field hospital, as I replaced some medical kit, the helicopter went into a steep dive. I fell forward with kit spilling all over the floor. I was terrified and convinced in that moment that I was going to die. After what seemed like an eternity but was probably about five seconds the helicopter levelled out. I managed to find my headset but when I put it on all I could hear was laughter. The pilots / a\*\*\*holes flying the Puma were having a 'bit of fun'. While they had fun I had the biggest sense of humour failure known to man. Ignoring the rank structure, I let them know what I thought of their joke when we landed. I was left with a deep hatred of flying though I am able to function as long as I can access pharmaceuticals. I take 10mg diazepam, which will help me relax and at least allow me to board the aircraft. I don't like having to take it but without it, I would not be fun to sit next to.

For a while our group chats nervously in Departures before splitting up to do some last minute shopping. I find a quiet area and start to watch a film as distraction from the impending flight.

After about an hour it is time to go to the gate where the group reunites. We board and find our seats. This is it; we are on our way.

I found out last night that Alessandro suffers with a fear of flying too after he was in an aircraft that crashed in South Sudan. I watch as he grips the arms of the chair with whitening knuckles. He is officially a worse flyer than me. In some kind of *schadenfreude* way it makes me feel slightly better.

The grim, somewhat austere airport in Casablanca is our halfway point. We have a four-hour layover here. The departure area is full of tired, bored people from many countries. There are a few non-governmental organisations (charities) represented here with lots of people heading to West Africa.

The highlight of Casablanca airport – which is devoid of all romance and there isn't a pianist in sight – is a lady called Julia who is an MSF psychologist travelling alone to Sierra Leone. She is going to work with the National Staff to help them through this awful time. She is a very kind and generous person who took pity on a hungry vegan (me) and gave me some fruit and nuts.

Before we board the flight from Casablanca to Freetown, our small group of MSF people exchange hugs. From that moment on we follow MSF's strict 'no touch' policy: 'Do not touch anyone, not even to shake a hand or put a comforting hand on a shoulder unless you are wearing PPE'. The no touch policy is both logical and slightly misleading. As an infection control policy it makes perfect sense and will help reduce transmission of the virus, it does however mislead people into thinking that you can get Ebola from touching a healthy person. No one objects however, we can all appreciate that it is meant to keep us focused and aware that things are different on this mission, and there are certain rules in place for our safety and that of others.

# Sunday, November 16

**Anna**
"Is there a doctor on board?" sounds over the intercom.

I awaken, startled. I had dozed off for a moment. I look towards Andy, who is sitting on the other side of the aisle. He's already standing up, and gestures to me to follow. I squeeze from my window seat past my neighbour and walk to the front, following Andy. It is half past twelve, the Royal Air Moroc flight from Casablanca, Morocco to Freetown, Sierra Leone, has been in the air for an hour. The plane is full despite the lousy timing of the flight in the middle of the night, and the Ebola affected destination. Many flights to Sierra Leone and Liberia have been cancelled due to Ebola. The remaining flights are very full.

In the middle chair of the row of three is a portly, elderly African gentleman. He has reportedly been taken ill. Next to him, trapped in the seat between the man and the window, is one of our non-medical MSF expats. She looks somewhat uncomfortable to say the least.

In normal circumstances, we would start with feeling a pulse, measuring blood pressure etc while trying to get some history from the patient. But circumstances are not normal. The main thing that is going through my mind is: 'Don't touch!' and 'Ebola?' Let's first just ask about his recent travel and where he comes from. The expat next to him realises that we are thinking about an Ebola diagnosis, and looks even more uncomfortable. The prospect of being trapped next to a potential Ebola patient on a flight is not one to relish.

With the help of the flight attendant, we get some information from the man. He says that he has lived in London for the past five months and that he has not had any fever. He had shouted out loud during a brief sleep, and had woken up a few minutes ago, in a sweat. By this time, he is feeling better. He seems to be doing fine. We decide on a pragmatic course and declare him to be healthy – at least for the remaining two hours of the flight. Perhaps it had just been a nightmare. Our expat colleague does not look overly comforted but is stuck where she is for the rest of the flight.

Walking back along the aisle I see almost all the passengers look in our direction with concern in their eyes. I nod to them to signal that everything is OK. It turns out we made the right decision. The remainder of the flight is uneventful. But any further sleep is out of the question for me.

We arrive at Freetown airport at a little past three in the morning, local time. We walk from the plane to the airport building in the dark, through a drizzling, warm rain. Two big buckets with taps, on stands, flank the entrance to the building; our first experience with the 0.05% chlorine water. Everyone has to line up to wash hands before entering the building. A uniformed employee makes sure no one skips this. We are all curious and smell the chlorine on our hands after washing. The novelty will soon fade, hand washing with chlorine will be a recurring ritual during our stay in Sierra Leone.

Inside there are extra checks. Everyone is handed a folder about Ebola and a form to fill in: where you are travelling from, where you're going to, whether you have any symptoms. After the usual line for the passport check there is a second line. A man in a white coat is posted behind a small table, armed with a thermometer, the kind that is pointed at your forehead like a gun. He checks the completed form and fills in my temperature, 36.7 degrees Celsius, so I can enter the country.

A short time later, we have collected our luggage, and are standing outside the airport building next to the office of the ferry service, which will take us to the capital. In the middle of the night, in the drizzle, we are transported by bus on the ten minute journey to the ferry port. The small ferryboats carry us in the dark across the bay to Freetown, a trip that lasts more than 30 minutes. Everyone's half asleep. At the other side of the bay, the group collects their luggage and gets into a couple of MSF Land Cruisers to travel onwards. Eventually we reach one of the MSF houses in Freetown at the break of dawn, around six in the morning. Everyone sits down on the couches, bone tired.

**Andy**

I am at the MSF Office in Freetown, it is six o'clock in the morning and I am worn out. Our group sits on the settees pretty much in silence now, the fatigue taking its toll. Kees the Finance Coordinator gives each of us an envelope with some Sierra Leonean money to see us through a few days and then we are travelling again. We have one final journey to the accommodation for our overnight stay before the trip to Kailahun. Sadly Alessandro is staying at a different hotel.

"It's because you're Italian mate, that's why you're not allowed to stay with us," I tell him. I am determined that we are not going to part in a civil and reasonable way. That said, we wave goodbye and climb back into the MSF vehicles to be ferried to our accommodation.

The drive to the hotel is amazing, despite my overwhelming fatigue. Everywhere I look people are out running, dozens of them, men and women of all sizes. "Is this normal?" I ask the driver to which he replies, "No, normally there are a lot more but ah, with this Ebola people are scared." I have not seen this anywhere in Africa before today.

We arrive at the Jam Lodge Hotel where we are served breakfast. Most people have omelettes but for Vegan Andy it's bread and jam. I am wondering if this is the mission where I go home thinner. On my previous three missions, totalling a year and a half in Africa, I have maintained every chubby pound.

I finally lie down on a clean soft bed about eight o'clock.

Ten o'clock and "Hallelujah" goes the cry, I snap awake. It is of course Sunday and the church next to the hotel is swinging into life. I try to sleep but even with headphones on I can hear "Praise be" and "Thank the Lord". I quickly surrender and rise from my bed. I have slept for two hours and it will be good to make something of the day.

Around midday I leave the hotel and head out for a walk with Julia and Monique (a Dutch nurse). We walk around 4.5 miles from the accommodation to Lumley beach in the Aberdeen district of Freetown. On the way we pass many people who wave at us and smile. One man spots the MSF logo on my bag and calls out, "MSF, you protect us from the Ebola virus, God bless you." It is very moving as he is a young guy who could have easily been more concerned with looking cool in front of his friends.

A short time later a young man called Noah approaches and asks where we are going. "To try to find a beach," I tell him. "I will take you," he replies, "It is a long way but the beach is very nice." Noah is selling balloons. He goes on to tell me that both his stepmother and best friend have died of Ebola. Noah walks with us all the way to Lumley Beach where I thank him for his help and commend him and his fellow Sierra Leoneans on their courage during the outbreak. "It's not courage sir, we have no choice."

Julia, Monique and I seek out some comfort albeit with a slight sense of guilt. We enter the air-conditioned luxury of the Radisson Blu Mammy Yoko Hotel and head for the veranda. Here we order a beer and watch the sunbathers roasting nicely as the children play in the swimming pool. We talk about the pleasure of a cold beer while contemplating the next month in unknown conditions.

In many ways life is just going on normally in the capital. There are however posters, billboards and reminders about Ebola everywhere. People seem to comply with the no touching advice. I know that this will be hard; Africans tend to go in for elaborate handshaking. As we relax in the hotel bar we discuss a potential long-term legacy from this outbreak. Is it possible that in this region the hand washing and hygiene education given during the Ebola outbreak could be built upon? So many people die from communicable and preventable disease due to poor hygiene.

A short time later we feel the sand under our feet. Lumley Beach is quite beautiful and we are happy to feel the warmth of the sun and hear the waves break on the shoreline. "Do you mind if we watch for a while?" I ask as we pass some teenage boys doing acrobatic flips from a wall onto the sand. Children play in the sea nearby, couples walk hand in hand and people drink at beach bars, all very normal. These familiar sights are punctuated here and there by billboards asking, "Do you know your HIV status?" and "Can you recognise Ebola?"

We decide to hail a taxi to return to the guesthouse, the sun is starting to go down and we have to follow the standard MSF security rule of not walking after dark. It has been a nice, relaxing day but I am tired now and will be having an early night tonight.

*Ebola in Sierra Leone*
There are posters and banners about Ebola everywhere, telling the public what to do if someone gets ill. Text messages are sent through mobile phone providers. Local radio stations frequently transmit Ebola songs, and give out information about what Ebola is, and prevention strategies. The entrance to all public buildings is flanked by containers of chlorinated water to wash your hands before entering.

The borders of the country have been closed. Regular citizens can only travel between the various provinces under strict conditions. Along the road, police checkpoints are set up, where they measure your temperature and where you wash your hands again.

During the time that we lived and worked in Kailahun (MSF had already been active there for at least five months) we saw a very positive attitude from the local people. The work of MSF was greatly appreciated in this district.

It is also important to realise that regular life in Sierra Leone continued, despite the restrictions and changes caused by Ebola. It is terrible that more than 14,000 people have fallen ill with Ebola in this country since the start of the outbreak, and almost 4,000 people have died (as per January 2016). But this is a country of about 6 million people, so 99.7 per cent of the population does not have Ebola. There are no big stacks of dead bodies on the streets in every city and village – an impression sometimes conveyed by some of the media at that time.

# Monday, November 17

**Anna**

We travel all day today. Kailahun is a remote province in the east of Sierra Leone, more than 400 km from Freetown. We've been picked up at our hotel at a little past seven in the morning. I've put on the white MSF T-shirt for the first time today. That makes me feel self-conscious, among all the experienced MSF-ers in the group, as if I do not deserve to wear it yet, that I have to earn that right first.

A few other MSF-ers from a different hotel are added to our group, including Alessandro, and so we leave Freetown with ten passengers and two drivers in two cars: a pick-up truck for the luggage and a passenger van. The road between Freetown and Bo is excellent, tarmac all the way, and recently built by a South Korean firm. This road was supposed to go all the way from Freetown in the West to Kailahun in the extreme East of the country. However, work ceased with the outbreak of Ebola when the South Korean company hastily withdrew its team. We pass several police checkpoints, where our MSF logos act as a free pass. The local population is not allowed to pass the district borders before nine in the morning, because of Ebola, and after that time only by special permission, so several times we pass a long line of waiting cars and trucks. At one or two checkpoints we do have to get out of the van, and get our temperature taken with the help of the by now familiar 'temperature guns'. At noon, we stop at the MSF compound in Bo, the location of another MSF EMC. Half of our group, including Alessandro, will remain here. The rest of us have lunch before travelling onwards, after a 'no touch' goodbye to our colleagues.

The first two hours after Bo are comfortable as the road is still tarmac. I'm in the front seat next to the driver and have a wonderful view of the countryside. A green, rolling landscape is all around us, with mountains in the distance. The road is often empty. When we approach a village or town, the number of motorbikes increases. Many of the motorbikes have one or two passengers on the back seat, and sometimes an incredibly large amount of baggage: cans of palm oil, stores of firewood etc. Even more abundant are people walking along the side of the road. They walk in a steady rhythm, used to going long distances, their luggage gracefully carried on their head. At some points, the walkers take a turn away from the road, onto a narrow trail leading in the direction of their village or home, which makes it seem as if they are disappearing into the jungle. I find myself looking in every direction; everything is new and overwhelming to me. In Kenema, we pass an EMC run by the International Red Cross. The driver slows down for a moment to point this out to us, and I strain to catch a glimpse with professional interest and curiosity. All I can see is a collection of large white tents and small huts. Not long afterwards, the tarmac road comes to an abrupt end, where work on the road has stopped due to the Ebola scare. We are on a rough soil track from here onwards.

An hour or so later, after having changed cars, I'm in the back of the first Land Cruiser, together with nurse Monique from The Netherlands and doctor Laura from the USA. In the front seat, next to the driver, is Canadian nurse Nathalie. In the pick-up truck behind us, Andy is seated next to the driver. A red soil road passes through thick green foliage and small villages, where the MSF Land Cruisers attract a lot of attention. The many potholes and bumps in the road cause me to fly up and down on the seat, in the back of the car, and several times I narrowly avoid hitting the roof with my head. The time is nearing half past four, and for the last hour the road has worsened so much that even the experienced MSF-ers call it a bad road.

I'm trying to hold onto my seat when suddenly the driver hits the brake. In front of our car, a Land Cruiser from the aid organisation Save the Children is halted. The cause of this is quickly clear. A local truck is stuck in the mud. The road is narrow at this point, flanked by thick foliage on both sides, so only pedestrians can pass. We get out of the car. It is nice to be able to stretch my legs. The expat from Save the Children tells us that she has been stuck here for the last hour. A group of people is at work trying to get the truck moving. We are in luck. Shortly after we arrive at the scene the men manage to get the truck out of the mud. They manoeuvre it to the side of the road, enabling our Land Cruisers to pass. Not long afterwards, we meet another stranded truck. This time it is an MSF supply vehicle and it has been stuck for a day. A rescue operation is underway. Again we are lucky, the road is wide at this point, and with some careful driving we can pass. This is the only road into Kailahun. Fortunately the wet season is at an end and things should improve soon, hopefully.

**Andy**
As we bounce through the potholes on the final leg of the journey from Freetown to Kailahun my mind drifts to South Sudan. In 2008 I was working in the country that was yet to vote on its independence from Sudan. I was working with MSF setting up clinics at Sakure and Gangura near the border with the Democratic Republic of Congo (DRC). Due to security concerns the decision was made that we would drive two hours to one clinic or two and a half hours to the other, work for about three hours and then return to base. This may seem like an inefficient use of resources but MSF takes security very seriously and it was judged that it was not a stable enough situation to remain in the clinics overnight. We therefore endured the 'road' four to five hours a day Monday to Friday. In the wet season, we would get stuck in the mud every other day or so and have to dig out the Land Cruiser, returning to base covered in red mud from head to toe.

I contemplate these and other events as our vehicle pitches from pothole to pothole, this time in Sierra Leone. The sight of the Land Cruiser in front breaks my sombre mood. Inside I see Anna bouncing about like a skittle on one of the parallel bench seats in the back. Her startled expression and the clear discomfort combine to make a very amusing sight. I am a bad person!

We arrive at the MSF Base in Kailahun about five thirty in the afternoon and are greeted by chlorine hand washes and temperature checks. We then proceed to the office to meet a few people and to be shown where our accommodation is located.

This is a hotel complex mainly on one level but with one building that is two storeys high. My room is small as hotel rooms go but for me it is luxury. It has a double bed and an en suite bathroom. There is a shower; it has a rather pitiful cold water flow but it works. I have never seen the like on an MSF mission. My accommodation in South Sudan in 2013 was a mud brick tukul (hut) with a tin sheet roof. The mud brick part was OK but the tin sheet was a nightmare. In the dry season it was like the 'cooler' in which the Germans locked Steve McQueen in *The Great Escape* while in the rainy season even a light shower sounded biblical.

There is a good reason that MSF has gone to the trouble of finding such accommodation for us and it isn't that they think we deserve comfort. The nature of the mission dictates that we must be segregated for infection control. No shared hygiene facilities and the ability to isolate any one of us were we to become sick. What starts as a pleasant surprise ends with the harsh reality of an Ebola mission.

We spend the rest of the evening in briefings with Bill the Project Coordinator (MSF speak for the boss!) and various other coordination staff. About ten o'clock I finally have a chance to Skype call Tracey and Mum and Dad to let them know that I am all right and to test the communication. We have Wi-Fi here, which is great but it is satellite based and therefore weather dependent.

*The MSF Ebola management centre (EMC) in Kailahun*
The EMC in Kailahun has been built on what was jungle, leased from its owner; it was built over a few weeks at the end of June 2014. The patients are housed in twelve big tents, eight stretcher beds per tent making a ninety-six patient capacity. The paths and areas between the tents are covered by corrugated sheets to offer some protection against the sun or heavy rain. Each zone has its latrines and shower huts. The latter are small empty huts where patients can give themselves a bucket wash. There are multiple water taps, connected to an underground pipe network, especially constructed for the EMC. Water is transported to the clinic in big trucks every day. Some of the taps are for drinking water, others for 0.5% chlorine water. This higher concentration of chlorine (0.5%) is used for decontamination of objects and PPE. Each tent also has a container filled with 0.05% chlorine, the diluted concentration that is used for hand washing. In every tent there is a table with a small supply of thermometers, pens, tape, diapers, and disposable cloths. Empty buckets are widely available for patients to use in case of vomiting or diarrhoea, or for cleaning purposes. Another essential item in every tent is a clock, which staff use to ensure they do not overstay the one hour maximum in High Risk.

Each area is segregated by orange plastic fencing, with an extra barrier between the 'suspected Ebola', 'strongly suspected Ebola' (also known as 'probable Ebola') and 'confirmed Ebola' areas. In order to reduce risk of transmitting infection we only ever move from a lower risk area to a higher risk area, never the other way around. Passing from one area to another we walk through a footbath filled with chlorine water, to decontaminate our boots.

Within the High Risk zone, there is an area where convalescent patients can sit and relax together. Sometimes, it looks like a busy terrace. A big board, painted white, has been constructed just outside the orange fencing, which can be used to project a film in the evening when the equipment is available.

At the back of the High Risk zone is an area where patients can receive visitors. Chairs on both sides of the orange fencing allow family and friends to sit down near to their loved one, with a safe distance of about two-metres in between.

Other items in the High Risk zone include a small hut where pregnant women can be separated from the other patients for delivery. There is also a mortuary, where deceased patients are kept until they are collected by the International Red Cross burial team.

The Low Risk area flanks the High Risk zone. At shift change, scrubs and boots are handed out at the entrance and this becomes a very busy and congested area, as all the staff vie for the correct sizes. Property lockers are located at the entrance and all personal possessions are left here. When we have our scrub suit and boots we go to the changing room.

Once dressed, we enter the Low Risk area. This part of the EMC contains the store and pharmacy, where we can get clothes and flip-flops for patients, pens, medicines, thermometers, bottles of drinking water etc. There's also the laundry, where a group of women wash the green scrubs and decontaminate the white boots by hand before putting them out to dry in the sun. There are also two tents for the laboratory where the blood tests for Ebola are carried out.

The medical team has two tents. The team consists of nurses, nursing aids, Community Health Officers (CHOs) who provide basic medical care in the community in 'normal' times, and doctors. Inside the tents are registers and patient files, some medical textbooks, a medicine cabinet, needles and syringes etc.

Further on past the medics area there is a big tent for the 'WatSan' (water and sanitation) team. This is a large team of people looking after hygiene, decontamination, sanitation, cleaning, and the safe removal of deceased patients to the mortuary.

At the border of the High and Low Risk zones are two dressing tents. These contain all the things needed to dress in PPE. There are multiple mirrors to check yourself and a large white board to record the name, entry and exit times of all the people working inside the High Risk zone. Personnel called dressers help us to don the PPE. At the other end of the clinic are two undressing tents. That is where we remove the PPE, helped by the 'undressers'. Four young men or women each shift have the sole task of helping the people coming out of High Risk to undress safely.

The ambulance entrance is located at the edge of the High Risk zone, near the dressing tents. Patients are assisted out of the ambulance and into the triage area. The driver can then take the empty ambulance around the perimeter of the EMC to the vehicle decontamination area.

A soil road runs along the length of the EMC. This separates the clinical and the non-clinical areas of the EMC. On the non-clinical side of the road is the area that is officially called the "unknown risk" zone. In other words the risk of contracting Ebola is probably as big or small as anywhere else in Sierra Leone. You work in your regular street clothes in that area. It contains the carpentry workshop, the patient kitchen and a big supply tent. There is a small hut for the National Staff health clinic, flanked by an even smaller hut serving as a waiting room.

Near to the health clinic is a collection of tents that is called 'the Hotel'. This is the area where discharged patients are received, and where, if necessary, they can spend a couple of nights waiting for transport back home. By the Hotel there is an area used by the 'health promoters' to conduct interviews and counselling sessions with the discharged patients.

Finally the expat canteen where we take our breaks. This area has been named 'Auntie Margaret's' after one of the local nurses who died earlier during the outbreak.

The day is divided up into three shifts for the National Staff: from eight in the morning to two in the afternoon, from two in the afternoon to eight in the evening, and a night shift from eight to eight. The expats work two shifts: from half past six in the morning to two o'clock in the afternoon (the earlier start in the morning shift in order to perform one of the most dangerous jobs: drawing blood for the Ebola test) or from two until eight in the evening. At night, an expat is on call in case the staff run into problems. Every shift, the expats enter the High Risk zone three times, if needed four times. They try to ensure that the National Staff do not have to go into High Risk more than twice, because the National Staff have been carrying out this work for over five months already whereas the expats are on a four to five week rotation.

# Tuesday, November 18

**Anna**

Christine, the American nurse and Medical Team Leader of our project, has us in her charge this morning. We start off with a number of briefings: about safety protocols, working and living in the base hotel, the EMC and finally the town of Kailahun. Once the briefings at base are complete we take our first trip to the EMC, a half hour's drive in an MSF Land Cruiser over an uneven soil road through the centre of Kailahun town, and on towards the Guinea border. Christine walks us around the EMC, including the outside perimeter of the High Risk zone, to give us a first impression of our new workplace. Under the burning sun, my white MSF T-shirt is quickly covered in sweat marks.

At noon, there are four of us in one of the two dressing tents: Andy, Laura, Nathalie and I. This will be our first experience inside the High Risk zone. Eliseo will be our guide. He is a very experienced Italian nurse who has often worked on MSF missions and has already worked in EMCs in Guinea and Liberia during this outbreak. He has been in Kailahun for more than a week now, and that is a lot in these circumstances.

We are dressed in green scrubs and white boots in the so-called 'Low Risk zone'. There is activity all around us, but it is hard for me to discern any pattern. So I decide to concentrate on the task at hand: to dress up safely in PPE, as we were taught in Amsterdam last week. We put on blue latex-free gloves. The yellow plastic overall, which we zip shut before sealing the zip with a stick down flap. Immediately, the temperature rises. The orange face mask that covers mouth and nose. A white hood over my head and shoulders now leaves only a rectangle free around my eyes. A dresser helps me to fasten the hood and hands me a heavy grey plastic apron. Someone asks me my name and writes it on the white hood, across my forehead. That way, my colleagues and the patients will know who I am. A second person writes a number on the sleeve of my overall, to keep track of me for the records. I put on a second pair of gloves, this time tight-fitting surgical gloves with long sleeves. Then the final step, safety goggles to cover my eyes and my glasses. These are adjusted carefully to cover every bit of my face not yet covered by the white hood.

It takes fifteen minutes to complete this procedure. I already feel the sweat running down my back. I have to control my breathing behind the face mask, and try to ignore the constricted feeling. I have to resist the urge to put up my hands to the safety goggles to check whether they are still okay, as this is more likely to cause a breach in the PPE rather than to improve things. All this while we are still standing in the safe environment of the dressing tent. The experienced dressers cast a critical glance at the newbies. We also check each other as we were taught last week to ensure that no skin is left exposed. Finally, Eliseo inspects us, his charges. Green light: we can continue onwards.

We walk in the direction of the High Risk zone in single file. Eliseo opens the gate in the orange plastic fence, walks in, stepping in and out of the chlorine footbath, and hands the gate to the next person. We follow his example one by one. The final person closes the gate. First through the zone with two tents for patients who are suspected of having Ebola but who are still waiting for their test results. A group of children between three and ten years old is playing in the opening of the first tent. Eliseo gives them a friendly greeting but calmly continues. Another gate and footbath and we are in the second zone: two tents for patients in whom the diagnosis Ebola has also not been confirmed yet, but where the diagnosis seems even more probable. Eliseo lets us glance inside one of the tents. Eight stretcher beds, five of which are filled by patients. The other three patients are sitting on plastic chairs in the area between the tents, which also has a covering made out of corrugated metal sheeting, planks and shade cloth.

I'm starting to get increasingly hot. Breathing is difficult and feels unnatural in this heat, through the face mask. My vision is limited through both glasses and goggles, although I'm relieved that they are not fogged up. I don't have any energy left to talk or to think much, I need it all to stand and walk, at a slow pace. Eliseo keeps a close eye on us all the time, to see that we are still OK. We pass through another fence, and another chlorine footbath. This brings us to the part of the EMC with the eight tents for patients with confirmed Ebola. In the first four tents are the patients who are most ill. A few of them have fled from the heat inside the tents and are sitting in the pathways between the tents. Or are lying down on mats on the ground. A small child is sitting next to his mother, who is lying down. We have to walk carefully to avoid stepping on anyone or anything.

I'm getting more and more hot and sweaty. I feel I can no longer stand it. As we were told, I speak up. "Sorry guys, I think I have to go out."

Eliseo moves over to me immediately. He looks straight into my eyes. Dressed up in PPE, that is the only way to make contact with someone. Despite the multiple layers of protective clothing, it is a strange, intimate kind of contact.

"You are finished? Good that you let us know," Eliseo tells me. We are near the exit to the undressing tents. "You move over that way, and they will help you to get undressed."

"I'll be fine. You go on," I answer him, putting on a brave face. Eliseo ignores this, and accompanies me all the way to the undressing tent, as is the protocol.

The undresser knows that this is my first time, and takes good care of me. He gives me step-by-step instructions, and stops me when I move too fast. Ten minutes later, at the end of the procedure when I am at the final hand wash, I thank him gratefully. I move away to a stool near the medical tent. It feels like a defeat that I was the first who needed to leave the High Risk zone while the rest carried on. I think I managed around half an hour and that is even without doing anything! What will happen when I have to start work inside High Risk tomorrow? Will it be too difficult for me? Have I travelled all the way to Kailahun for nothing?

My fellow expats try to comfort me. Everyone has a story of how the first time was the toughest. I am praised for giving a timely warning that I needed to get out. But that is scant consolation.

## Andy

After our first foray into High Risk we rehydrate, have some lunch and then Anna and I take a five-minute walk down the road to the graveyard. It is a tragic and sobering place. Many people are buried in marked graves however some are unidentified and will remain so. We are told that MSF is currently in discussion with the International Red Cross who are conducting the burials, regarding the standard of their work and the failure to mark the graves clearly. It seems unimaginable that people who have lost their loved ones should have their grief compounded by the anonymity of a badly organised graveyard. Anna and I say little, we just stand for a while absorbing the scene. After five minutes, I turn to Anna and ask, "Shall we go?" To which she replies a simple, "Yes." We are moved by what we have seen. This is a valuable experience for us. It demonstrates how the people of the area have suffered over the last six months and it makes it clear that we need to be considerate to everyone involved: local population, patients and the staff of the EMC.

Back at the EMC we meet up with Laura. Together we walk to the road barrier that governs access to the facility. Here, some local entrepreneurs have set up small stalls to cater for the staff of the EMC, which has rapidly become one of the biggest employers in the area. We like the look of some oranges but debate the safety of buying fruit that will have been handled by others. I am initially against the idea though the oranges do look rather juicy. After much discussion we ask the lady to put the oranges in a plastic bag for us. We will wash them in chlorine inside the bag before peeling them. In retrospect the length of the discussion is mildly comical. I have never deliberated the purchase of citrus fruit in quite such depth and it is unlikely I ever will again.

Our first day at the EMC has been overwhelming. The sheer number of patients (77 at this time), the severity of their illness, a system which is new to us, the large number of National Staff to get to know and a graveyard that clearly demonstrates the tragedy that this outbreak has brought to Kailahun.

*How the diagnosis Ebola is made*
It is often difficult to differentiate between Ebola and other diseases common in Sub Saharan Africa, such as malaria, especially at an early stage of illness. In order to decide whether a patient should be admitted to the EMC we use a list of agreed criteria, which include symptoms such as fever, muscle aches, bleeding, and also include possible exposure, such as attending a traditional funeral, ill relatives or preparing bush meat. If a patient has a lot of symptoms that could fit with this deadly viral haemorrhagic disease, or he has some symptoms plus potential exposure, he will be admitted as a 'Suspect Ebola' case or a 'Probable Ebola' case, depending on clinical judgement.

Every patient that is admitted is tested for Ebola by a blood test. If the test confirms the diagnosis, it means a move to the 'Confirmed Area'. In the case of a negative test what happens depends on the circumstances. If the symptoms only started one or two days before admission, the test might be falsely negative because the virus level in the blood is still low, so the test is repeated two days later (while the patient remains in the 'Suspect Area'). We also do a repeat test if we have a strong suspicion that the patient does have Ebola. Only if the test is negative and clinical circumstances fit with this, is the patient discharged as not having Ebola.

In the evening, we newbies are introduced to the team back at the base. I sit there waiting for my turn to introduce myself. Should I try to be funny? Should I play down or just state previous experience? I always hate this bit. No one is listening anyway. If I can judge people, the staff just want to relax and eat their dinner. I make it snappy and think it went OK. Once we have all said hello we can relax and enjoy the food. It looks like there will be vegan options for me here though it may be very limited in variety. That's not a massive problem for me, I am easily pleased.

# Wednesday, November 19 – Starting work

**Andy**

I get up at half past five in order to leave the house at six. We drive to the EMC as the sun starts to rise in the East, the Sierra Leonean morning is quite beautiful. There are a lot of people around already, women preparing food, children playing or returning from the forest with wood for cooking fires. As we pass, the children cannot resist shouting, "Pumweh, Pumweh," (white man) at us. I am sure that this will become the soundtrack to each day here. In Uganda it was "Mzungu" or "Muno" and in South Sudan "Kowaja". I smile at my new name.

Arriving at the EMC we greet the staff who are about to finish the night shift. It has been a long night for them and they still have an hour and a half to go. Despite this they smile and welcome us to work.

Eliseo and I start the day with blood sampling (venepuncture). We take blood for two main reasons: one is to confirm the presence of the Ebola virus, the second is to assess a known positive patient, as to whether he has cleared the virus and is ready for discharge. "Blood sampling is the most dangerous thing," Eliseo explains, "if you get a needle stick injury[1], you will die. No one survives it, because of the high load of virus."

---

1 Needle stick injury: where the needle you have taken the patient's blood with, accidentally penetrates your own skin.

I ask Moses, one of the National Staff from the night shift, if he would mind coming into the High Risk area to assist in the blood sampling by acting as a sprayer (everything we touch is sprayed with 0.5% chlorine and we wash our double gloved hands in it too). Moses is tired but willing to help with one last job.

Eliseo explains the system to me, how we work methodically from the Suspect area through the Probable area and into the Confirmed area, never going back as it could transmit infection. I listen keenly to everything he says.

In Low Risk we prepare everything to take the samples, we gather the equipment, label the blood tubes and bags. Finally we write a list of the patient's location for each sample required. We then move to the dressing tent and prepare for our entry to High Risk.

Eliseo takes the first three samples. They are tricky, as the patients tend to be quite dehydrated and their veins are hard to feel through two pairs of gloves, and even harder to hit with a needle. "I can see that this is very difficult mate," I offer by way of encouragement to him while wondering how I will fare.

Eliseo manages to collect one blood draw and the other two samples he takes as finger pricks, much the same way as diabetics do to test their blood sugar. Two samples are from young women who are reasonably stable, the third is a little girl who is frightened and doesn't want to come to us. We approach her and Moses explains what we need to do. I don't understand the words but his tone seems caring and gentle. We sit her on Eliseo's knee, Moses continues to talk soothingly to her as I prick her finger and milk a sufficient quantity of blood into the tube. In the end the girl is very brave.

I take the final sample in the Confirmed area. I am nervous though I have taken hundreds of blood samples in my career. In England we treat every sample as if it is from an infected patient (although more likely with HIV or hepatitis than Ebola). Even with that in mind this is different.

Moses has called over the young man that I'm supposed to gather the sample from. The patient sits down in the plastic chair. I sit down in the chair in front of him, having made sure that I have my equipment all ready: a sharps safety box on the floor to my right, the tourniquet, blood tube, needle etc. But there is too much distraction going on around us. This is not a sterile hospital setting. A few children who are well on the road to recovery are playing nearby, running in and out of the tent. A man sitting just outside the tent has a radio and is playing loud music. I ask Moses for help, and he moves the playing children to the other side of the tent, and tells the man to turn off his radio for a minute. Moses then returns to help me. I make sure he knows what he is supposed to do, before I unsheath the needle and guide it into the vein in the young patient's arm. I know that I have hit it straight away. Moses hands me the tube, I attach it to the adaptor and it rapidly fills with blood. As soon as I have enough blood, I remove the tourniquet, place a cotton wool ball at the ready, and remove the needle from the patient's arm, to put it straight into the sharps box.

Trying to feel a vein through two pairs of gloves, goggles affecting my vision, the fatigue of being in the PPE nearly an hour and the warning about needle sticks ringing in my ears combine to make this a blood sample I will never forget. This is the single most satisfying sample of blood I will ever take.

## Anna

A little past nine in the morning. I am inside tent C3, the tent with confirmed Ebola patients who are moderately ill. I have entered the High Risk zone with Konneh, a very experienced local nurse, and a hygienist to help out as a sprayer. After yesterday's quick retreat I worry whether I will be able to do better today. It is still early in the day, so the temperature is still moderate. That is a help. I'm standing in the corner of the tent, a very slight fog on my goggles, but easily enough vision to read and write. Konneh is kind and is quick to notice that he should not expect too much yet from this newbie expat.

I will be recording the observations and clinical assessments of the patients this morning. Someone has come up with a clever way to get notes from the patient rounds in the High Risk zone into the patient files located in the Low Risk zone because, of course, nothing at all can be taken out of the High Risk zone. Before entering the High Risk zone, I fill in the patients' name and number in the columns on a sheet of paper. The medical clerk photocopies this, to keep one copy for himself, and one for me to take with me. Every tent has a supply of pens that stay there.

Skilfully, Konneh puts a thermometer in the armpit of the first two patients, and starts to ask questions of the woman in the first bed. He translates the important things for me.

"She hasn't vomited anymore, though she does have diarrhoea."

I try to find the entry for 'diarrhoea' on the paper, which is marked with a table. Every column represents a patient, every row a symptom or sign. I can't find the row for 'diarrhoea'.

"Muscle aches, painful joints," Konneh continues.

I find the row for muscle aches and place a mark in the patient's column. Finally I spot the diarrhoea row.

"Temperature 38.1." While Konneh is already moving on to the next patient, I quickly scribble down my notes on the paper. I need all my concentration to follow Konneh and note down his remarks. Everything done in PPE uses up a lot of energy. I still struggle to think for myself or make a spontaneous suggestion. I'm just glad to keep up, for both tents C3 and C4. Konneh makes sure we finish exactly within the allowed hour.

At the orange fencing separating the High and Low Risk zones, Sylvanus, the medical clerk, is waiting to receive the data we have gathered, paper and pen in hand. Every symptom on the list has a number so you call out across the fence to the clerk: "Patient 1060, temp 36.6 - 1, 4 and 5" instead of "Fatmata Kargbo, temperature 36.6, muscle aches, diarrhoea and vomiting." Or "Patient 1102, temp 38.3 – 1, 4, 5, 9, 10, given extra pain medication," and so on. This reduces the chance of miscommunication and is also better from a privacy point of view. The clerk records it on his paper. When you have called out all the information on your paper to the clerk, you throw away your copy, and move on to the undressing tents to free yourself from the PPE. When you reach the medical tent, you'll find the clerk's notes, ready to be transcribed to the individual patient files.[2]

This time when I leave the undressing tent, wet through from sweat despite the fact that the sun will not reach its highest point for a while, I feel relieved. I have been able to stay in for an hour, without fainting! The next time I enter the High Risk zone that morning shift, I notice that I have improved even more. I even have enough energy left to help some patients to drink. This gives me confidence that I will be able to get used to it.

### Andy

Bokarie, one of the National Staff Nurses, and I enter tent C2 where there are six patients. The sickest is a young man called Kai. I remember his name as we had a member of staff in Leer Hospital with the same name. Kai is very much in the prime of his life but there is no doubt in my mind that he is going to die. Bokarie and I approach him and can clearly see that he is struggling to breathe with a respiratory rate of more than 30 breaths per minute. He struggles to swallow water or Oral Rehydration Solution (ORS) due to pain in his throat as well as nausea. His disease process is too far advanced for him to survive.

Bokarie explains to Kai that we need to try to give him a drink. "I'll sort out some medication, if you can give him a little fluid," I say to Bokarie. We will not be

---

[2] Several months later, MSF started using an iPad in a special plastic cover, which could be decontaminated, for the purpose of recording patient notes in the High Risk area.

starting an intravenous drip, as it will make no difference to his outcome. I open the plastic bag that I have prepared and take out a syringe with morphine and one with metoclopramide. I return to the bedside and ask Bokarie to explain to Kai that I will be giving him a couple of injections. The morphine will help with both the pain and hopefully his anxiety to a degree, the metoclopramide is to help with the nausea. Just after I give the injections the poor man vomits over both Bokarie and myself. We clean him and reassure him that the medication we have given should help but it will take a little while. We spray chlorinated water onto both the vomit on the floor and our aprons before going to the wash point for thorough cleaning of our gloves and other PPE. I think to myself, PPE is life. This young man's body fluids are teeming with virus and one mistake could mean infection.

    I turn back towards the patients inside the tent and contemplate the tragic scene of suffering that lies before me. I only hold this thought for a moment as it is our job to do what we can to alleviate the situation and we are very much working against the clock. Bokarie and I walk to the bedside of a little girl who we were asked to assess by another team. She is nine years old and very sick. Tragically, she is also alone. She was crying out as we saw Kai. I asked Bokarie what she was saying and he told me "She is calling for her mother." When we finally get to her she is very weak and only able to manage a few sips of ORS. She is soiled and needs to be washed. Bokarie turns her gently from side to side as I wash her and change her diaper. It is clear that the movement causes discomfort so again we administer pain relief. It is so upsetting to look into these people's eyes with the knowledge that they are going to die. Other than to keep them comfortable we are very much limited in our options. The interventions we can do merely support the patient to try and prevent death from an avoidable cause such as dehydration, malaria or treatable infections. As yet there is no Ebola specific treatment that we can administer.

*Neglected diseases*

The lack of a specific treatment for Ebola makes it one of many 'neglected diseases'. Which could be retitled 'diseases that affect only the poor'. No significant investment goes into research for these diseases and where treatment does exist it is often out-dated and potentially toxic.

Human African Trypanosomiasis (Sleeping Sickness) for example. Many of the drugs used to treat this disease were developed in the 1960s. One drug that is used in the latter stages of the disease has a 30 per cent failure rate and 5 per cent of those given the medication are killed by it.

There is talk of Ebola vaccine development, indeed trials have already taken place. It could be suggested that the rush to develop a treatment is based on self-interest. The pharmaceutical companies with their advanced Research and Development projects are now being asked to concentrate on Ebola by governments whose populations have had a taste of Ebola albeit in a very small and contained way. The fact that a poor Sierra Leonean, Guinean or Liberian may benefit seems very much incidental however altruistic it makes politicians feel.

# Thursday, November 20

**Andy**

I am on the afternoon shift today and at two o'clock I enter the EMC and change into scrubs. I wander through to the Low Risk area and greet the morning staff. I am looking at the coordination board (a white board with a drawing of the tent locations with magnetic markers that show patient location) when Mohammed, one of the administration staff, approaches me. In a low, clearly saddened voice he tells me that both Kai and the little girl I cared for yesterday have died this morning. Dreadful news to start my shift and it will take me some time to collect my focus.

I am working with Pria, a Finnish nurse, today. We have a brief chat about the sad events of the morning and then take the full handover from the morning staff. It is now late in the afternoon and I am finishing in the Dressing tent and fully kitted in PPE I am ready to enter High Risk. Janet, one of the Sierra Leonean medical staff, and two hygienists accompany me. Anna was supposed to go with us, but she has been re-tasked to meet an ambulance arrival. The plan for this hour is to move newly confirmed Ebola patients on stretchers from the Probable to the Confirmed area. This is incredibly hard work in PPE. Any kind of physical exertion is draining but carrying a stretcher while ensuring safe footing is rapidly exhausting. One of the patients will need an intravenous cannula when we arrive in tent C4 as she needs a drip to deliver rapid rehydration. The cannula insertion is difficult because of fogging in my goggles but I manage to hit the vein first time. I set the drip on full flow and then immediately leave as my facemask is starting to move in and out with my breaths. This is a sign that it has become saturated with moisture from expired air. Once wet the masks lose their efficiency as a barrier.

It is a relief when I get to the undressing station as I know I am going to be out of the PPE in about ten minutes. The jet of cool chlorine water hitting the outside of my suit feels great even though it is a pretty noxious solution.

Leaving the undressing tent I walk to the medical tent and sit for a few minutes while drinking half a litre of water. I drink three to five litres of fluid per shift; three litres in a morning shift, more if I am working in the hot afternoon.

In the afternoon Pria and I sit and work on some administration. I feel sorry for her, she has been here for a month and leaves next week but she has had a skin reaction to some horrible little insects called Nairobi Flies (Paederus beetles). These little monsters are attracted to the EMC lights. They drop down onto the people below who then, as a reflex, swat them. When crushed on the skin they release a toxin, which causes inflammation and a reddish rash. The rash develops into blisters. Somehow, the Nairobi flies have a preference for dropping down onto Pria. The bad news for her is that if we have any broken skin, especially to the hands, wrists, face and neck – the least protected areas in PPE – we are not allowed in High Risk and cannot do the job we came to do. Also, the blisters will sometimes leave permanent scars, and the last set of blisters is on her forehead. I chat to her quite a lot as the shift progresses. I feel it is important to stress to her that the work she has done here has made a significant contribution to the project.

**Anna**

Afternoon shift. The dressing tent is crowded at half past four in the afternoon. There is a bright hot sun in a clear blue sky. The tent's shade offers only limited relief from the heat. But the atmosphere is good, we joke around while putting on the PPE. We are a large team: two local nurses, two sprayers, Andy and I. We have made a clear plan of action for our time in the High Risk zone, to make use of every minute in PPE. But you need to be flexible here. I'm halfway through dressing in PPE when we get the news that an ambulance has just arrived. There are no other medics available at the moment. An extra sprayer is quickly asked to dress up and help me to deal with the ambulance. Andy and the others will carry out as much of our original plan as possible without me.

So as soon as both of us are in PPE, Emmanuel, a young sprayer, and I walk to the left, in the direction of the ambulance. A white Land Cruiser has been parked under the corrugated sheet roof of the reception area. The driver is impatiently waiting for our arrival. He is safely seated in the front of the Land Cruiser, separated by a fixed partition from the patient area. He is under instructions not to leave his seat until the ambulance is unloaded.

Emmanuel picks up the container of 0.5% chlorine that is always at the ready near the ambulance entrance and carefully sprays the back doors of the vehicle, from top to bottom. Then he sprays a big wooden block. We pick this block up together and set it down at the back of the ambulance, as a step for the patients. Emmanuel then sprays my gloves.

I open the first of two back doors of the ambulance. That is the moment you can see who is inside the ambulance, how many patients and the condition they are in. It is very rare that patients arrive with any kind of documentation. It's a moment to brace yourself to expect anything.

This is an ambulance from the Kailahun province itself, which has arrived without warning. It carries only one patient, a woman of about 30. I gesture to her to remain seated for a moment. Emmanuel now sprays the inside of the door. We repeat the procedure with the second door. Only then do we ask the woman to climb out. I help her step down on to the wooden block, and support her during the brief walk to the triage hut where she can sit down on one of the many plastic chairs. Meanwhile, Emmanuel closes the ambulance doors. The Land Cruiser can now drive off around the EMC to be decontaminated.

The triage area is a wooden building with a roof made out of corrugated sheets, it is shaped like a long, narrow rectangle. Two orange plastic fences have been put up in the middle, along the whole length. One side of the hut is in the Low Risk zone, the other in the High Risk zone. Between the two fences, there is a 2m wide no mans land. Triage is the gateway between the ambulance entrance and the patient tents.

My colleagues at the Low Risk side carefully throw the woman a bottle of water and a packet of biscuits.

They start to interview her, to find out who she is, where she is from, what her symptoms are, whether she has been in contact with an Ebola patient, etc. I stand at her side, still in PPE, and take her temperature. Emmanuel has finished his work on the ambulance and joins me.

But before we are ready to move on, there is more news: another ambulance has just arrived, this time from far away. Now that the Ebola epidemic in Kailahun itself seems to be more and more under control, a large number of our patients these days arrive from other parts of the country, from holding centres in Makeni, Tonkolili or Freetown, hundreds of kilometres to the west. Every morning, our Medical Team Leader phones these holding centres to tell them how many beds we have available, and how many patients they can send. The ambulances have to travel the same long road that we took to get here, sometimes six to eight hours along bumpy sand roads filled with mud and holes. I know what it's like to travel them when you are feeling well – let alone when you are feeling ill and nauseous. And these ambulances won't stop for lunch or toilet breaks along the way. It must be a hellish ride. They usually don't arrive at our EMC before the end of the afternoon.

Emmanuel and I go through the whole procedure again, and I open the ambulance doors. This time, the sight that meets my eyes is horrible. This ambulance is packed with nine patients: five children between three and twelve years old and four adult women, one of whom is clearly in an advanced stage of pregnancy. Most of them are obviously ill. They are cramped from the hours spent in their packed position. One by one

I help the patients climb down from the ambulance and support them on the walk to triage. The youngest child, a girl of about three years old, I have to carry in my arms, because she is too ill to walk or to sit. I have to support her head, to stop it from lolling back. The last patient in the ambulance is a young boy of about 11 years old, who is also too weak to walk. Emmanuel and I carry him on a stretcher for the 10m to triage.

We have only just put down the stretcher when we find out that the last ambulance of the day has also just arrived. Emmanuel and I look at each other: what shall we do? Do we have enough energy left to handle a third ambulance? We decide that we have sufficient reserves. Emmanuel closes the doors of the second ambulance, and together we move the wooden block to the side to make room for the new ambulance.

By this time, Emmanuel and I are a practised team. This ambulance contains five men and a teenage boy, who can all walk themselves to the triage hut, with some support. We have been at work in PPE for about an hour now. It is warm, I start to get less quick in my thinking. I feel it is getting near my time to leave. I signal to Emmanuel, and together we walk away, leaving behind the 16 patients who have just arrived, some in chairs, a few have lain down on the floor. I can't manage to take their temperatures, someone else will have to do that. I can't even look after the three-year-old girl, or the eleven-year-old boy, who are both clearly very ill. I hate it, it's tragic, but it is too hot now, I have to leave them behind.

The two of us walk the whole route through the High Risk zone to the undressing tents at the other end. The undresser guides me safely out of the PPE.

That gives such a feeling of relief, freedom, especially taking off the by now moist face mask. The green scrubs are wet through from sweating, even my hair is wet. First I have to sit down and drink some water and oral rehydration solution (ORS), which we always have around. By this time, it's about six o'clock, the temperature is starting to drop. It may still be about 27 degrees Celsius I think, but not the bright sun of the early afternoon.

About half an hour later it has turned dark, and I have recovered somewhat. I change into a dry pair of scrubs, and go to help out in the triage hut, on the Low Risk side. It's a big job to collect the needed data from all the patients, to determine whether and where to admit them. We also want data on their home village or town, and how they may have caught the disease, which will help in efforts to prevent the spread of the disease. Some patients don't have the energy to call their answers across the 2m of no mans land. But these are important data in a large outbreak.

The three-year-old girl turns out to be accompanied by two sisters: one four-year-old and a twelve-year-old. The two sisters are not ill, but apparently have been put in the ambulance just because no one knew what to do with them. We can try and get some information on the sisters from the twelve-year-old only that's not easy. She probably has not understood everything of the tragedy that has happened to her and her family in the last few days or weeks. She says that both of her parents have had Ebola, supposedly they have survived, but the girl doesn't know where they are. Nor can she tell us where her three brothers are. She is carrying a note that contains the phone number of an aunt, and that's all.

These are tricky cases: it would be good to keep the three small sisters together, so that they can support each other, but if we admit the eldest two, who do not show any signs of Ebola, they will run the risk of contamination. The girls, of course, run a high risk already of having contracted Ebola through contact with their parents, their sister, and now through the hours of travelling in a packed ambulance – so they will have to be watched carefully for the next 21 days. We decide to send the two girls to the 'hotel' across the road. They can spend the night there, before being taken to the special Ebola orphanage tomorrow.[3] We hope someone can find out where their family is tomorrow, and where they would be best looked after.

The three-year-old will have to remain behind in the EMC by herself: she is very likely suffering from Ebola. A difficult situation: she is too young to look after herself, even if she was not this ill, and now she will not have any family in the clinic.

---

3   The Ebola orphanage in Kailahun is run by the government of Sierra Leone. Children under 18 years old who have survived Ebola and are discharged cured from the EMC but who have no adult relatives, are looked after there, until living relatives can be traced who will take them in. In a separate house, the orphanage can also take in children who have not had Ebola themselves, but who are abandoned or left by themselves because of Ebola. The latter group of children have often been in close contact with the disease either through their relatives or in a holding centre or ambulance, so for the first 21 days after their arrival they are watched carefully for development of any signs of disease.

It's eight o'clock before we have figured out what to do with all of the 16 new patients who arrived this afternoon. Everyone on the staff is tired and upset by the suffering. The patients still need to be taken to their beds and given medication. A long day.

**Andy**

I have been in this job a long time, nearly 20 years and I have never worked in a more heart-breaking context. Taking the two little girls to the hotel is so sad. Knowing that they have already lost so much and now they have to wait to see how their sister will fare.

This evening, I walk from my room to a large tower in the centre of the base. There is a function room at the bottom and then some stairs, which I climb. At the top of the stairs I walk to the external wall of a recreation area. Here I can appreciate the view of the surrounding area. I can see the neat line of MSF Land Cruisers near to the main office to my left. Over to the right the lush green forest looks quiet and beautiful, birds flit from tree to tree inside and out of the base compound, they are truly without borders.

It is six thirty and the sun is starting to set. I have admired sunsets all over the world and certainly won't be the first or last to find it relaxing and a time for contemplation. I mull over the first couple of days in Sierra Leone and hope that I can settle into the job quickly and can cope with life and death in the intense environment of the EMC. Just after seven o'clock the sun dips over the horizon and I head back to my room.

*Admitting a patient in the EMC*

The process of admission is long and tiring for the patients. Once they are out of the ambulance, patients either lie on stretchers or sit on plastic chairs in triage separated from the EMC staff by two fences that run in parallel with a 'no man's land' in the middle. This is a good infection control measure but a nightmare for communication. The patients are weak in both body and voice. Taking their medical history is therefore difficult. We gather information about their symptoms and potential contact with Ebola patients, to determine whether they fit the case definition of Ebola, and to decide whether they will be admitted to the 'Suspected' or 'Probable' area, or in rare cases discharged directly.

Once the triage is completed, medical staff in full PPE go in to the patients. As part of the admission an all-important wristband with the person's name and number is put on. This is vital as it is very easy to lose track of people in the busy EMC. Also, many of the patients are unaccompanied children. They are walked or carried to their assigned tent. The newly arrived patients are handed a blanket, a mat, soap, a towel, a toothbrush and toothpaste, and if needed, fresh clothes. They are then given the first doses of the standard supportive medication which includes antibiotics and antimalarial drugs. We do not test for malaria due to the inherent risk in pricking fingers to test blood in an Ebola outbreak. We cannot conduct lengthy investigations to look for infection sources and these patients in their weakened state are more susceptible to other infections. It therefore makes sense in this context to treat everyone for malaria and with a course of antibiotics. The medication also includes a painkiller and vitamins.

An important aspect of admission is an explanation of hygiene matters. The Staff carefully explain the no touch policy in the EMC. They tell the patients not to share food, plates or toiletries, and also explain the use of water and chlorine water.

**Anna**

It is past nine before I am back at the hotel this evening. I'm very tired, and have trouble balancing on one leg at the entrance to the compound, while the sprayer sprays the soles of my shoes one by one – a routine procedure, even for me, by now. Ah well, I turn it into a joke. The first thing I do on my return to my room is take off my sweaty socks (which never really dry out for the whole of a shift after you have been in the High Risk zone in PPE) and put on different shoes. Luckily, we were warned at the Amsterdam training to bring lots of socks and underwear. I also take off my old glasses and put on my newer ones. That is a kind of ritual exorcism. Apart from the socks and underwear, my glasses are the only personal thing I wear underneath the PPE inside the High Risk zone. It should be safe, covered by the safety goggles, but still it feels good to wear a different pair of glasses when I'm 'at home' in the base hotel. Just like the hair band I wear underneath the PPE: this goes into the bin every day. A bit overdone perhaps, but it feels like the right thing to do.

Then, it's time to get some dinner, with my malaria prophylaxis. And the day ends with a meeting of the expat medical team.

# Friday, November 21

**Anna**

In the past few days, I have started to suffer from a nasty cold with a sore throat. A souvenir from the Netherlands undoubtedly made worse by last weekend's tiring journey. Yesterday evening, my voice had almost completely disappeared. It has been decided to change our schedules so that I can have my day off today instead of next Sunday, and I can get some rest and recuperate. Otherwise, I would have had to leave for work at 6 o'clock this morning for my next morning shift.

So today I take it easy and stay in the hotel. I talk as little as possible, because my voice is still gone, but otherwise I'm already starting to feel better after a good night's rest. It is very frustrating: I've come here to work, I'm not really ill and there is such a lot to be done and now I'm just hanging around the hotel. But if I would really get ill, I would become a burden, so I had better take the time to get well. I fill the day with some reading, an afternoon nap, writing in my journal, and a Whatsapp conversation with my mother. She proudly sends me a video clip of her granddaughter, a photograph of my father working in the garden. All the kind of things that are usually so normal are such a contrast to the last few days here. She also sends me photographic proof that she has actually started on the knitting project to 'keep me safe from harm' – the first part of the green cardigan is taking shape.

**Andy**

After handover I pair up with Lois, one of our National Staff, and head to the dressing tent. I want to film the dressing process today so that people back home can understand. We stop at the hygienists' tent to find someone to come in to act as a sprayer and a pleasant guy called Stephen volunteers immediately. In the dressing tent I set up the camera, which is like a light to moths. Suddenly I am besieged by helpful staff wanting to assist me with dressing, asking me questions about patients and offering to write my name on my hood etc. I joke with the staff about them being Hollywood stars as I dress in my PPE.

All of our jobs on this first run into High risk are in the Confirmed area so we pass through the Suspect and Probable areas rapidly. Arriving in tent C5 I locate a baby whose mother died in the EMC last week. I sit him onto my knee and start to feed him with some therapeutic milk that we prepared earlier. "Come and see this," I call to Lois. When she arrives I point out how the baby is totally ignoring the strange yellow suit, the mask, the gloves and the goggles and is looking straight into my eyes. To think that a child can look past all of that equipment and spot the only true human feature and then cling to it is amazing.

I see another two patients in C5 but at the 45-minute point, I start to really suffer with the heat. I speak to Lois and Stephen apologetically, "I'm really sorry but we are going to have to leave. I'm struggling." They understand and we both walk to the undressing tent together. The rule is that you always stick with and look after your buddies.

Once I have rehydrated I take a walk round to see the convalescing patients who are accommodated in tents C7 and C8. There is a fence that separates their area from Low Risk and we have a table and chairs on the Low Risk side so we can sit and chat. Our psychosocial team uses this or another, more private area at the back of High Risk, where patients wouldn't be overheard by others for counselling. The medical people like to go there too sometimes to carry out assessments to see how people are progressing, other times for selfish reasons such as now. I sit on one of the chairs and watch as the patients play games, sing and talk. It is remarkable to see how relative normality can be achieved in such abnormal circumstances.

# Saturday, November 22

**Anna**
This morning, I do the rounds in tents C5 and C6, with Musa's help. Musa is a young Community Health Officer (CHO). He finished his training a few months before the start of the Ebola outbreak, and afterwards worked as a volunteer in a few government projects, because he couldn't find paid work. This work with MSF is his first paid job. He is intelligent, ambitious and very talkative.

In this part of the EMC, the rounds can be done in a different way. We do not need to dress in PPE as we do not actually enter the High Risk area, these patients have recovered sufficiently to walk up to the fence themselves. Musa and I are each sitting in our green scrubs and white boots on a small wooden stool near the orange fencing. The wooden box with the patient files is on a third wooden stool, near at hand. At the other side of the orange fence is the usual 2m of no mans land. In this case, a table fills this space, to make it easier to hand the patients on the other side their food and drink.

From our seats, Musa and I can see about 20 patients seated randomly in the open space in the shade of the roof. Against the second orange fence, at the inside of the High Risk zone, John has put two chairs. John is a teenager who has been in the EMC for a while and who has nearly recovered. He is patiently waiting out his days until his Ebola blood test will become negative and he can go home. He has spontaneously taken on the role of our helper during the rounds. As soon as he sees us walk up with the box of patient files he gets into action. He sits down on one of the chairs, next to the bucket with chlorine and the cup filled with thermometers. Musa greets him cheerfully in Mende.

I pick up the first patient file. "Fatmata Kargbo," I call out.

"Fatmata Kargbo," repeats John. A young woman in the background gets up and walks towards the empty chair next to John. Musa and I exchange a friendly greeting with the woman, and Musa asks her in her own language how she is doing. Meanwhile, John hands her a thermometer which she expertly puts into her armpit, underneath her T-shirt. Musa translates her answer. "She still has some joint pains. Her pain medication helps a little, but not enough. She can eat, and is no longer nauseous."

"And does she still have diarrhoea?" I ask.

Fatmata understands my question before it is translated, and shakes her head. I promise her that I will increase the dose of her painkillers. The thermometer beeps. She gives it to John, who calls out the result across the fence. "36.5." Good. Fatmata has not had any fever, vomiting or diarrhoea for the last three days. I will put her on the list to have her blood drawn tomorrow morning to repeat the Ebola test. If it is negative, she can go home.

"Mohamed Koroma," Musa calls for the next patient. John repeats the name, but it takes a while before we see a reaction. Three small boys appear in the opening of the tent. A boy of about 12 years old pushes two smaller boys of four and eight in front of him. Mohamed turns out to be the youngest of the three. He is very shy. John has meanwhile routinely decontaminated the used thermometer with chlorine. He hands each of the two smaller boys a thermometer and helps them to place them under their arms correctly. Thankfully, the boys are doing well. The eldest of the three has been declared cured and fit to leave two days ago, but when we wanted to discharge him, he protested. He wanted to stay to look after his little brothers, who would otherwise be on their own. We are not really sure whether they are blood relatives, but we don't care. Of course we allow him to stay.

In this way, we see every patient one by one. This is a much more relaxed way of working than in PPE in the High Risk zone. We have time for a joke, and a chat. These are the people who will make it. They have turned the corner.

Death however is never far away. Just as we are finished and stand up to walk away, a pick-up truck passes that has just picked up the bodies of deceased patients from the mortuary, to take them to the graveyard. All patients at the other side of the fence rise from their chairs too, out of respect for the dead.

## Andy

On this, as with most MSF missions, we work six days a week. I am off duty today and intend to spend the day relaxing. I wake around half past seven and wander over to the dining hall. As ever I wash my hands in 0.05% chlorine water and then enter. Taking a seat next to Laura I suggest that we go for a walk after breakfast. There are no major security concerns in the area and we are allowed to walk in pairs as long as we have a phone with us and obey bio-security rules – no touching and no going to crowded places such as markets.

We leave the base about half past eight and head down the road away from Kailahun Town. We pass through a number of villages on the way and are warmly greeted by the inhabitants who have long since accepted the presence of MSF and the odd looking people that work for them. The people have been exposed to a lot of education about Ebola and infection control. This is made clear to us as we walk through the villages and children approach us. The older kids stop the youngsters from rushing over and grabbing us. "No touch, no touch," they tell the little ones.

It is very green here and quite lovely, rolling hills on all sides and off into the distance we can see some large mountains. Banana and papaya trees are everywhere as well as what I think are coconut trees, which are apparently out of season at the moment, either that or they aren't coconut trees at all which would also explain the absence of coconuts! I may have spent a year and a half in Africa but I seem to have failed dismally when it comes to knowledge of the continent's botanical riches. I ask Laura, but she too has no idea. "It's a good job we can do a bit of medical work as we are pretty useless otherwise," I comment as we leave the possible coconut trees and press on.

About one hour from base Laura quite rightly advises that we may be pushing the limit for distance from our base, I reluctantly agree and we turn back.

Ludicrously we have forgotten to bring any water. "I guess we are getting to like that lovely dehydrated feeling already!" I suggest.

By the time we arrive back at base, I am as thirsty as I am leaving the High Risk area. I wash my hands at the main gate and have my temperature taken, my shoes are then sprayed with chlorine. Only then am I allowed to enter the compound. I walk to the office, which is the hub of the project. Here the epidemiologist, logistics, administration, medical and management teams carry out their planning and reporting. The office also has a very important resource – two big fridges full of cool refreshing water. I make a beeline for the fridges and grab two bottles. I down the first one in about 30 seconds flat and then collapse into a chair and chat to Jenn our Aussie epidemiologist. She has a warm smile and a friendly personality; this combined with a great sense of humour makes for a very nice colleague and I enjoy talking with her as I rest and enjoy the drinks.

In the evening I take a walk over to the dining area about six o'clock. Laura and Nathalie are already there and Ann and Jenn soon join us. The young lady serving the food (one person does this per day and has theoretically been trained in food hygiene) is morose in the extreme. It has become my goal to make her smile each time she is working and today is no exception. She slops some green stuff onto my plate and I watch as the vegetable oil separates from the food and forms an orange moat around my meal. Before she adds a scoop of rice I tell her that she is looking very beautiful today. She immediately becomes a different person, a big smile forms and her demeanour changes entirely. My work here is done and I take a seat feeling satisfied.

# Sunday, November 23

**Andy**
I am on an early shift today. I have been allocated a team of about ten medical staff who rotate on a roster. My team is on the early shift today, which means that I will be responsible for coordinating their activities. I have never aspired to be in management, my passion lies in direct patient care but accept this role is part of the job when working with MSF. I suspect that my dislike of the coordination role is to blame for the atrocious night's sleep I had last night. I have been awake since quarter past four when I woke from a dream about infection control.

Ann, a very pleasant English nurse, Laura and I are now en route to the EMC. The driver carefully negotiates the potholes in the dirt road through the town. We pass the mosque followed by one of the many churches. Even at six o'clock people are up and about starting their working day or cooking breakfast near the roadside.

At the EMC, the shift starts with blood draws as normal (if anything here is normal). I enter High Risk with Ann and manage each of the eight blood samples I am to take. It is nice to begin the day with direct patient care.

After the blood samples are taken I am supposed to allocate the newly arrived day staff to the various roles.

However, I start as I mean to go on and call over Sheku, one of the senior National Staff medics. "Sheku, you know these guys and what they are good at, I want you to do the allocations, please." This works in a number of ways: it gives Sheku some responsibility, it genuinely makes the best of people's skills and finally it gets me out of at least one job I really don't want. I don't mention the latter out loud.

Once the allocations are done I go to review the patients in the convalescence area. It takes me a while, as there are many patients. Mostly they are doing very well. There are two with high temperatures to whom I give paracetamol and I will check them again in a couple of hours. I ask one guy about his appetite and he tells me through the interpreter that he is eating very little and he has no appetite. The others start to laugh. "What's so funny?" I ask. Through the laughter they tell me that he has double portions at every meal.

After about an hour, I leave the fence bordering the convalescence area and walk past the laundry area and the upside down wellington boots drying in the sun. I meet Ian, the Canadian scientist who works in the small lab tent where the Ebola blood tests are analysed. It is midday and he is about to go to the medical tent to present the results. I walk with him and along with Russ, one of the doctors, we go through the test results and are pleased to see that some of the patients in the convalescence area are now ready for discharge. I feel especially happy as I have just been talking to them and know how desperate they are to go home.

I spend the next 30 minutes or so tracking down each member of the medical team who carried out the rounds this morning. I ask each for a briefing on the state of the patients that they have seen. I will be handing over to the afternoon shift at two o'clock and I want to complete that handover in an informed way.

At two o'clock, I start the handover, one minute later I am apparently finished as Laura steps in front of me and starts to hand over the people she had seen earlier. The others follow suit and I am now standing at the back totally sidelined. The expat nurse in charge of the afternoon then starts to allocate the jobs for the late shift. I am somewhat surprised that she doesn't ask me about the transfers and discharges or in any way interact with me about the morning shift. I exchange a knowing glance with Anna who has watched this unfold; I seethe quietly and then walk away. I survive the shift albeit with a mild ego bruising. I guess people have differing personalities and differing standards of courtesy.

**Anna**
Afternoon shift again today, so the morning off. The largest part of the morning is nice and cool, about 23 degrees and a fresh breeze. But when the sun comes out at the end of the morning, the temperature rises quickly. I spend the morning quietly reading. And something else: checking the first proofs for my debut novel, which my publisher has just sent me by email. It is supposed to be published early next year. I can hardly wait. It is quite a contrast: correcting proofs of a novel about a revolution in a Dutch town in the 18$^{th}$ century, before going on duty in an Ebola hospital in 21$^{st}$ century West Africa.

We are in luck today for food: Eliseo has a day off and he loves to cook. He spends a large part of his day in the kitchen with the female kitchen staff, and produces some wonderful meals, considering what he has to work with. All food is either cooked in big pots over an open fire, or grilled on a wood-stove barbecue. Today, we have an Italian risotto and a fresh fruit salad for lunch. A very welcome change from the usual chicken twice a day, with white rice or spaghetti and one of three different spicy sauces, only occasionally accompanied by some fruit or vegetables.

On our way to the clinic today, the streets are crowded. A lot of families in their Sunday clothes are walking along the roadside on their way home from church, the women and girls in beautiful dresses in bright colours. Muslims and Christians live together peacefully here, the city has multiple small mosques and churches. There's a busy market going on in the centre of town.

Handover at two o'clock, where I see that Andy, who is trying to lead the proceedings, as is his task today, is completely sidelined by some other expat staff. They don't even notice anything amiss. I send Andy a commiserating glance – things are too busy to do more at the moment. The white board of patients is pretty full, with a lot of patients that could use extra medical attention.

The heat is intense when I enter the High Risk zone in PPE around three o'clock in the afternoon, accompanied by a National Staff nurse and Fajah from the WatSan team as my buddies. This time, my task is a so-called ORS-round in tent C3 and C4. ORS, or oral rehydration solution, is a combination of water with salts and sugar. It is better than pure water to supplement fluid loss, although it doesn't taste great.

The patients have all been instructed that drinking ORS is of life and death importance. Because of the vomiting and diarrhoea an Ebola patient can quickly become dehydrated, especially in the African heat. The sick patients are often too weak and lethargic to put in much effort themselves, even to leave their beds. So we visit each bedridden patient, to help him up and to put a cup of ORS to his mouth. And another. These ORS-rounds are a fixed part of every shift. While you are in there, you are able to check on the patients at the same time, and give them extra medication for pain or nausea if needed. We also check to see if they have had diarrhoea, and change a diaper where necessary. Fajah keeps an eye on us, to make sure we work safely, and cleans up vomit on the floor, or sprays our hands in between patients.

This ORS-round, my most memorable encounter is with Osman, a little boy of nine years old, from Bombali District, about 200 km north west of Kailahun. He is very ill. His father is on the bed on the other side of the aisle, also very sick, too ill to get up, let alone to look after his son. But he is clearly worried about him, and when we enter the tent, he asks us to help his son first.

I squat next to the boy's stretcher. He is lying down on the bed, exhausted, his eyes closed. Some dried blood on his lips, from his bleeding gums. I help Osman to sit up in bed, my right arm supporting him underneath his shoulders, and put the cup of ORS to his mouth. Slowly, he drinks a sip, and another sip. Then he wants to lie down again. But I keep at it, and keep talking to him, to make him drink. Very slowly, sip-by-sip, the boy drinks half of the big cup. That is all that he can manage, this round. I am glad that he doesn't vomit it out again immediately. Carefully, I put him down on the bed again. I ask Fajah to decontaminate my hands and apron with his chlorine spray and then I move on to the next patient. I emerge from the PPE around four o'clock, drenched in sweat. Time to drink ORS myself.

An hour later, it is time for another round in the High Risk zone. This time, to help two National nurses to transfer some patients. A considerable number of patients are to be moved from the 'Probable Ebola' to the 'Confirmed Ebola' area because their test results have come back positive. This is very traumatic for them, of course, the confirmation of the diagnosis. Our mental health counsellors have already broken the news earlier that afternoon.

It is more difficult than it sounds to do these transfers, hampered by PPE, when there are so many patients, even though they are all able to walk. We carry a list of patient names and numbers. At the corresponding tents, we call out the patient names. Every patient carries his or her few personal belongings. Most people only have a toothbrush, toothpaste, soap, a blanket and a mobile phone.

One of the patients suffers from schizophrenia. He has caused us problems multiple times already in the past two days, especially at night. He tends to become agitated, and refuses to listen to reason. The orange plastic fences are not able to hold back people who deliberately want to leave. It is not easy to explain the necessity of staying put to a man suffering from a paranoid delusion. We are trying to calm him down with the right psychiatric medication, but that is difficult and it takes time. The man needs to be firmly encouraged to walk along with us.

The other patients follow us more easily. But a young man of about 20 years old complains: he manages to explain to me that he thinks that someone made a mistake, that he is not supposed to be here and that he wants to be with his brother and sister. Luckily, one of the nurses happens to know that the man's brother and sister are in one of the 'confirmed Ebola' tents, so we can reassure him that after the move he will be able to visit them whenever he wants to. Bobor, a ten-year-old boy, starts to cry inconsolably after we have moved him to his new tent, and we can't make out the reason. We assume he is feeling ill and misses his family, both of which we cannot help.

In the middle of all this, another nurse in PPE asks my advice. He was sent into the High Risk zone to prepare a patient for discharge because she has been declared cured. But the woman refuses to leave. She wants to wait for her three grandchildren, who are still in the clinic. The children are luckily on the mend, but they are not yet ready to leave. The EMC is pretty full, there are not many empty beds. The nurse wants me to decide what to do. I tell him to let the woman stay. The children can use her help and support, and I know she has lost at least one son to the disease, so she has been through a lot herself. She is not the only one who stays on in the clinic for a few days although cured. I already mentioned the 12-year-old boy looking after his two brothers, and there's the mother of a six-month-old baby, who is waiting for her child to recover.

I have another encounter with the boy Osman during this round. While I'm visiting his tent, I try to get him to drink some more ORS. This time, he is much more clear-headed, and he can sit up to drink the complete cup. Perhaps there is some hope for him.

Back in the Low Risk zone, when we have rested a bit, it turns out that we will be able to solve Bobor's problem as well. In the transfer of patients we apparently wrongly left one patient behind in the 'Probable Ebola' area, by accident, although she was on our list: Bobor's mother! The boy was too upset to explain this to us, and the mother was too shy to speak up. A stupid mistake, we can only blame it on the heat, and the PPE, and the large number of patients. We make sure mother and son are reunited as soon as possible.

# Monday, November 24

**Andy**

As the song goes, 'what a difference a day makes'. Also what a difference colleagues make. I am working the afternoon shift with Kenichi (a Japanese paediatrician) and Anna. I am coordinating but will make sure I get to do some clinical work too.

At three o'clock I go to the dressing tent with Sheku. We have a clear plan of what we intend to do. It is simple and vital – hydration. We are going to pass straight to the Confirmed area with the intention of helping a number of patients who have been flagged up as struggling to drink.

We arrive in tent C1 and approach an elderly man. He watches us but does not move. Like many other patients, he is extremely weak and uncomfortable. Ebola patients suffer both severe joint pain and sore throats and it feels almost cruel when we sit them up and push them to drink. We know however that this is vital if they are to survive. "I am sorry," I say as I help him into a seated position. He can barely acknowledge me but as we offer the water with dissolved rehydration salts he tries hard to drink. He manages a few millilitres before it is clear that he is unable to take any more. I suggest to Sheku that we try again in a few minutes after we have seen a couple of the other patients.

We move to the opposite side of the tent to see a very sick 11-year-old boy called Lamin. Again, he is alone.

Illness is often an isolating state but in a context such as this, even more so. Each of the patients is wrapped up in their own Ebola journey and is either too sick to interact or sleeping due to severe fatigue. There is therefore little communication between the sickest patients in the EMC. Sheku and I sit Lamin up and give him a drink of ORS. He manages surprisingly well though he complains of a sore throat. I offer him something for the pain, which he manages to swallow with difficulty. I talk to Lamin for a while. I ask him about his family and about school. He tries to answer but talking is painful for him. I ask Sheku to apologise for my making him talk when his throat is sore. We leave him to rest, hopefully the pain killers will help soon.

It would seem obvious that if someone were struggling to drink, we would set up an intravenous (IV) drip to support his or her fluid intake. In this context however, intravenous rehydration is avoided where possible. This is due to the danger of inserting cannulas (the needle via which the drip is given) and also the risk of life threatening bleeding if the cannula were to be dislodged when the patient is unmonitored. Yesterday, Christine, the Medical Team Leader, made the decision that we are not to use the intravenous route for rehydration at this time as it is proving impossible to monitor the safety of the infusions. A couple of nights ago, she had to come to the EMC about three in the morning as a psychotic patient was trying to leave the High Risk area and walk out of the EMC. This would of course cause a massive infection risk and so was a significant problem for her to deal with. While she was inside the High Risk area, she found an intravenous fluid bag that had fallen to the floor, while still attached to a patient; this had backfilled with a litre of blood, which could have killed the patient.

In addition to this physical risk there is another dimension that we had to consider. At various times in this outbreak wild rumours have circulated, ranging from 'Ebola not being real' to 'the white men want to kill you or steal your blood'. The last thing we need is backfilled IV bags that seem to confirm this notion. For these reasons it was decided that we will focus on intensive oral rehydration until a safe approach for intravenous fluid delivery is determined.

**Anna**

A week after our arrival in Kailahun, I've been assigned an extra task, starting from today: the responsibility for so-called 'National Staff health'. It is usual in MSF missions for the organisation to provide care for everyone, both local population and staff. In this Ebola mission, we provide a general medical service for the employees (though not for all of their relatives). This is because we want to encourage employees who become ill, possibly with Ebola, to report quickly, to provide treatment and prevent the spread.

A small hut in the area across the road from the EMC is the designated staff clinic. Employees can come in for a walk-in office hour if they are feeling ill, or have injuries. One of the CHOs, Karimu, runs this clinic. He also looks after the discharged patients in the hotel tents, until they travel home. I will supervise him from now on. When Karimu has a day off, like today, things are done differently.

When someone needs to be seen in the staff clinic, they shout across the fence to the medical tent in the Low Risk zone of the EMC, and one of the expat doctors walks over to the staff clinic. If I am on duty, this will be my task.

This extra task also comes with an extra mobile phone, a number that National Staff can call day and night if they get taken ill. This is meant primarily for suspected Ebola. Another of my new duties is to keep in touch by phone with National Staff when they've been potentially exposed to Ebola (without PPE) until the 21 days of incubation are over and we know they have not been infected. At the moment I have a list of six names to call once every few days to ask them whether they are still feeling well, or are running a fever.

This afternoon, I'm only called across to the staff clinic once. In the waiting room I find a 21-year old man from Kailahun who works in the Outreach team as a 'health promoter' – the people who travel to the villages to educate the people about Ebola, and to gather information.

I invite him over to the staff clinic. This has been especially designed with Ebola in mind. In the middle of the small square hut, two fences of the familiar orange plastic have been put up, separated by a metre of no mans land. The patient sits down on the other side of the fences from me. I carefully hand him a thermometer, without touching him.

"What's wrong?" I ask him. He speaks enough English to do without a translator.

"I have a fever, since yesterday. I also feel very tired, and I have lost my appetite," he replies.

Concerned, I ask after other symptoms. He does not have diarrhoea, there's no vomiting. He does report muscle aches and he can't sleep. His family at home is not ill, and he has not visited a funeral recently. He is not aware of any unsafe contact with an Ebola patient. The thermometer in his armpit beeps: 38.6 degrees Celsius.

Not good. This could be Ebola. While I'm starting to consider how I will get him safely to the EMC across the road to get him tested, he finally comes out with the most important piece of information. Proudly, he tells me that he is an Ebola survivor. He has been a patient in our EMC himself this September, for 22 days. He fully recovered, and afterwards joined MSF. As a survivor, he is well qualified to explain about Ebola and what happens inside the EMC, and how important it is to come forward when you are ill.

Having had it once, he can't get Ebola again so it is safe for me to walk over to him, crossing the fences to examine him. This doesn't give me any extra information. If his fever is not caused by Ebola, then it is most likely malaria. That's very common around here. We are not able to do any diagnostic tests in the staff clinic, not even a malaria test, so I have to decide based on his story. I hand him a full course of anti-malaria treatment, and tell him to report back if he doesn't get better in three days time.

I mentioned an extra mobile phone: MSF makes sure that every expat gets the use of a personal mobile phone that works on the local network. I haven't used it much so far. Once in a while, I receive a text message from the provider to let me know how much credit is left on the phone. Or a so-called 'EbolaMsg', sent to all users. For example on November 19: "If you're feeling sick, get help quick quick! Early medical care can increase your chance of surviving Ebola." Today: "If someone is sick or suspected with Ebola, do not touch, call 117. While you wait for help, offer the sick person as much fluid as they can drink." A very smart way of reaching people, mobile phones are very common here.

Home on time today, driving back to base directly after the eight o'clock handover. After dinner, a short meeting in the dining hall, primarily to introduce the new expats who arrived today. This includes two new expat nurses so, believe it or not, when they start their work in the EMC the day after tomorrow, we, the four medics who started last Wednesday, will no longer be the least experienced people in the EMC.

Online I receive news from my hometown Nijmegen. In my hospital back home, the Radboud University Medical Centre, a patient has been admitted who has just returned from Sierra Leone, and is suspected of having Ebola. Weird thing to think about. I know exactly how the safety protocols will have been put in place again and how my colleagues in Nijmegen will be dressing in PPE under completely different circumstances. I send them a message to wish them well with all the extra work.

*Outreach*
Another important part of the MSF Ebola project in Kailahun is 'Outreach'. A number of expat nurses head a large group of National Staff, who again are in touch with hundreds of local volunteers throughout the province. They have all been taught about recognising Ebola, and

what to do if someone falls ill. They are MSF's eyes and ears in the many small towns and villages in Kailahun, and they report any suspect circumstances. All deaths should be reported as well, of any cause. When a death is suspected to have been caused by Ebola or there is a suspicion of someone with Ebola being kept hidden, an MSF team is sent to the spot. The Outreach team also keeps in touch with local chiefs and traditional healers.

When someone from Kailahun is admitted to the EMC, the Outreach team visits his home village, to educate the villagers and to trace any contacts. The Outreach team also take the patients back home when they are discharged cured. This helps to let his neighbours know that he really is cured and no longer contagious.

# Tuesday, November 25 – Death

**Andy**

I have already been into High Risk this morning for the blood draws. During my second visit to High Risk it is ten o'clock as we pass by tent C1. Eliseo says, "Let's just look in and see if anyone needs hygiene." Diarrhoea afflicts many of our patients and they are too weak to walk to the toilet. We therefore carry out regular hygiene rounds supplemented where possible by spot checks such as this. I enter the tent with Eliseo. "I'll check Lamin," I say and walk over to his bed. The boy is worse than yesterday, very lethargic. With the help of Sarah, our National Staff colleague, I sit him up to try a drink but it is clear he cannot manage and I am reluctant to push him too much. The danger of aspiration (fluids going into the lungs) is high and whatever we do, we do not want to do harm. Sarah and I lay him down again and settle him into a comfortable position on the bed. We then rejoin Eliseo who is just finishing with another patient. We briefly leave the tent before Eliseo goes back to collect some paperwork. "Bad news," he warns us upon his return, "Lamin has died." My heart sinks.

Lamin never got to grow up, fall in love and live his dreams. He is one of many. More than 300 people have died in the EMC since June. The difference is that I looked into his eyes and held him while we tried to give him a drink. I saw the care that was given to him and how the team suffers as they realise that he is not going to survive. We cope, people are resilient beings but it hurts.

When I finish undressing from my PPE, I walk to the convalescence area. People sit chatting, playing cards and recuperating before being discharged. I just sit and watch, sometimes we lose and it hurts but here at least I can see hope.

**Anna**
Around four o'clock, I enter the High Risk zone in PPE with Mary, an experienced expat nurse from the USA, who is visiting the project for a few days, and one of the national nurses. Our tasks include a visit to tent C1, to give some medication to a patient. On the first bed in the right hand corner is the body of the boy Lamin, covered by a blanket. Moving a deceased patient safely to the mortuary is a complex operation, and needs to be planned, so it sometimes takes a while before it gets done.

When entering a tent in the High Risk zone, it is good clinical practice to cast a glance on each patient inside, whatever the task you set out to do. Especially in the tents with the very ill patients, such as C1, because you never know when the next person will have time to visit. This time, we find out that the patient in the bed next to Lamin has also passed away. Sorrie was a 25-year-old man who was brought in by ambulance from the west of the country. He did not appear to be too sick on arrival at the EMC. He earned his living as a motorbike taxi driver. This is a common occupation. Cars are rare here and a motorbike can easily transport two or sometimes even three passengers. At the interview in the triage hut he had told us that he had not been in contact with any Ebola patients. But in his line of work he could easily have had an infected passenger on the back of his motorbike. Also, a lot of the patients, especially those from holding centres from the other side of the country, are ill and frightened when they arrive at our EMC. They are often afraid to tell us all, and think that they need to protect their family back home from prosecution and quarantine by not telling the truth. Just as Sorrie may very well have been infected by one of his passengers, he can easily have transmitted the disease to a lot of people if he still continued to work after the first symptoms started.

We lay out Sorrie's body, and cover him with a blanket. When we walk away from tent C1, we leave two dead patients underneath blankets, next to the living ones.

As soon as we leave the High Risk zone, we set things in motion to have the dead bodies removed to the mortuary by the WatSan team. I fill in the necessary papers for Sorrie: a form with a few details, name, age, his home village, and his father's name. The only phone number we have is his own mobile number. It will not be easy to get in touch with his family to let them know what happened. That is a task for the Outreach team. I also enter Sorrie's details in the death register, a large book with one line per death, and I note down his death in the general patient register. Finally, I write his name, patient number, age, gender and home village with a black marker on a small wooden stake, When the burial team collects the bodies from the mortuary, tomorrow or the day after, they will take these wooden markers with them to mark the graves.

It's almost six o'clock by the time I re-enter the High Risk zone, this time with a team of nurses, for an ORS-round. While busy dressing in the dressing tent – I'm already dressed in the yellow overall – I'm taken aside by Russ, the Canadian expat doctor. His in between shift of the day is ending, and he is about to leave for the hotel. He asks me to take a look at the patients in tent C4, while I'm inside. A nursing aide has just returned from the High Risk zone, after handing out food, and she had the impression that one of the patients in C4 was dead. This always needs to be confirmed by a CHO or an expat. A wry assignment.

I know the people in tent C4 a little by this time. They include little Osman and his father, and the young man who missed his brother and sister. On my way to the tent, dressed in PPE, I run through them in my mind: who will it be? Who will I find dead? When I arrive at the tent, a few of the patients are lying quite still. My goggles are quite fogged over this time, I see everything through a mist. So I have to bend closely over each patient one by one to see whether he or she is still alive. In PPE, it is nearly impossible to be certain about the presence or absence of a heartbeat by feeling the pulse, and I have to peer closely through my fogged-up goggles to be sure about a breathing movement. I resort to shaking the patients awake, to at least see some movement. To my relief, they all move upon my touch. It was a false alarm! As I've woken them up, I help them drink some ORS. The boy Osman is clearly doing a little better. He complains that he has already drunk such a lot that he doesn't want anymore. He asks for a radio. He still looks exhausted, but if he is starting to complain, he must be getting a little stronger.

Burials

Once every few days, a team of local employees of the International Red Cross drives to the EMC in a pick-up truck. They collect the death certificates and the wooden burial stakes. In the mortuary, they take the bodies of the patients who have died since their last visit, safely enclosed in a double layer of body bags. They drive the few dozen metres to the EMC's graveyard. This graveyard has been filled with hundreds of graves since the EMC's opening in June. The graves are very close together and have been dug in a haphazard way. Most are marked by simple wooden stakes with the patient details written in black marker pen. The markings are quickly fading in the African sun. Some markers only read 'DOA' – Dead on Arrival – and the date of arrival of the ambulance. In those cases, the name of the deceased has not been traced yet. A few of the graves have more elaborate markings. These are the graves of people who come from nearby towns or villages, where relatives and friends have been able to visit the grave already, and to leave a personal touch. To prevent the spread of Ebola, travelling between the various provinces has been very much restricted in Sierra Leone. The majority of the patients in the past few weeks are arriving from hundreds of kilometres away. It will be months before their relatives and friends can try to visit their loved one's grave.

# Wednesday, November 26

**Andy**

It sounds like it is going to be a busy afternoon for me today. Nathalie is handing over to us outside the medical tent. The whiteboard is full of magnet-backed disks with numbers representing patients. As she gives her report I scribble notes and highlight the more serious cases that I would like to see as soon as possible. C3 and C4 seem to have the highest concentration. This is a deliberate strategy by the team. We try to cohort the sickest people into one or two tents so that we are able to focus on them easily.

As soon as the handover is complete I head for the dressing tent with John, one of the National Staff medics and a hygienist to act as a sprayer. We are in a good mood as we dress. I ask John about his favourite football team and am mock disappointed when he replies, "Manchester United." I tell him that I am a Leeds United fan but he looks at me with a bemused expression. I guess Championship football isn't overly popular here. I try to tell him that they were Champions League Semi Finalists in 2000-2001 but I am wasting my time. "Ha, ha, I was five!" he replies and I change the subject. It is not until I put on my goggles, the final piece of my PPE, that I realise that my list of jobs is in my scrubs pocket – now covered by yellow overall and apron. John doesn't know how to reply when he hears me mumbling that I am an idiot,

I think he just accepted that as a given, possibly back when we were talking about football.

Fortunately, I know the sickest patients are in C3 and C4 and I know their names so I am sure I can locate them easily. We set off into High Risk and make our way to the confirmed tents. In C4, the father of the little boy Osman is sat on the edge of his bed and is responsive to us but clearly unsettled. He is working hard to breathe and complains of pain in every joint. He cannot find a comfortable position. I crouch next to him but as ever to the side just in case he were to vomit suddenly. "I will have a quick look at Osman and then I will get medication for you," I try to reassure him.

Osman is confused and unable to sit up. He cries out for his dad but he isn't able to be there for the boy as he is too sick. This must be awful for both the frightened little boy and the father whose instinct would be to protect his son. John and I sit Osman up and he takes a drink of ORS. He tells us that he too has pain so I administer analgesia to both him and his father before we have to move on.

In C3 there is a young man called Alimany. He is 19 and supports Chelsea: this is one of the first things he tells me. He says that he is a midfielder and he is a good player. His physique is consistent with him being a sportsman, yet his young body is teeming with virus and he will not survive. He knows it. "I die, I die," he says as we help him back to his bed after he has used the bucket by his bed to pass diarrhoea. We try to reassure him but we know he is right. The effort of transferring from the bucket to the bed is clear and distressing. John and I clean him properly before trying to give him a small drink. He complains of nausea so we give him an injection of metoclopramide, which should help.

We look in on a couple of other people in the tent. Then Alimany tells us that he wants to go to the toilet again. He wants to use the latrine and not the bucket. Of course he does, he is a 19-year-old man, his bed is next to a girl about the same age, and we have no screens. There is little dignity in Ebola. I probably should have said no to him and insisted that he used the bucket but I couldn't bear to add further indignity to this poor man's suffering. John and I therefore walk him to the toilet. It is a huge effort for all concerned. Alimany struggles with the effort due to his disease and John and I battle with the discomfort of PPE but it is worth it to give Alimany what he wants. He uses the pit latrine as John and I hover nearby. Once he has finished, I clean him and help pull up his Chelsea shorts. We then support him back to the tent. By the time we arrive he is in significant trouble, he is working very hard with his breathing. We lay him on the bed, sit him up so he can best expand his chest and after a few minutes he seems to settle again. We ease him back onto the bed and he is asleep almost immediately.

As John and I stand I notice that the young lady in the bed next to Alimany is is crying. She is clearly upset seeing him suffer, add to this the knowledge that she has the same disease. I have no idea how these people must be feeling, not even close. I try to reassure her through John but I feel like a fake. I will make a point of checking on her and will make sure that it is handed over to the other staff too.

I turn to John to say that it is time for us to leave High Risk; before I can speak, he points at my face: "Your goggles have slipped, I can see a bit of your face." That's a breach of my protective equipment, a definite reason to leave the High Risk area. In the undressing tent, I take a look in the mirror. About a centimetre of my face between goggles and hood has become exposed. I undress in the usual way but then I wash my face carefully in weak chlorine solution. It's only a minor incident, but I will report it anyway as we are asked to be totally open with anything like this.

Back at base I am once again frustrated with the communication situation. I have been trying to contact Tracey over the last few days but each time the Skype connection fails. This is infuriating as I am desperate to chat to her properly and to see how she is bearing up with my being away. It is often more difficult to be the one who is left at home than it is to be the one leaving. I know I am OK day to day but Tracey can only hope. We manage email messages but that is a poor substitute for hearing her voice.

**Anna**

Apart from all the Ebola misery, it is also difficult to provide good medical care to people who may not have Ebola. An unexpected ambulance drives up from a village not far from here, with one patient, a man of about 35 years of age, called Emmanuel. Expat nurse Ann receives the ambulance. The patient has to be carried on a stretcher to the triage hut. As usual, there is no documentation, and the ambulance driver only knows that the man has been found inside a house, and has vomited. Inspection from a distance of 2m across triage, and by Ann, standing next to him in PPE, reveals that the man is completely paralysed on the left side. It appears to be a recent paralysis, rather than a long-term condition. The man has to be supported when sitting up. He does seem able to drink water safely with a little bit of help. His temperature is 37.5 degrees Celsius, when measured axillary, which is just at the threshold of what we consider to be 'fever' in the case definition of Ebola. According to CHO Tommy, the man is very unclear in his speech. That's hard for me to judge in a different language. He does not really seem to have a lowered level of consciousness. We find no wounds or abrasions. We have no information about possible contact with an Ebola patient. What could it be? Perhaps a 'normal' stroke? But he is young for that. Severe malaria of the brain? But that usually leads to diminished consciousness or even coma. Ebola after all? He does not really fit the case definition, but we cannot rule it out with the limited information we have, and with someone who has a fever, has vomited and lives in this area. It is clear that the man will need a lot of nursing care, so if we decide it is probably not Ebola and send him to a regular hospital and we turn out to be wrong and he does have Ebola, he could potentially infect a lot of care workers. On the other hand, in our EMC we will not be able to give him optimal care for his paralysis inside the High-Risk zone, and he runs the risk of catching Ebola if he does not have it now.

In the end we decide to admit him, and to start the standard treatment, including anti-malarial treatment. It is clear that Emmanuel needs a lot of extra care: medication has to be administered under supervision to make sure he does not choke on it, and he has to be helped when eating and drinking. We worry that he will quickly develop bedsores on the stretcher bed, because he can hardly move himself. Repeated attempts to trace his family and get more background information have failed so far. With some effort, the man can tell us in his own language that his eldest brother is named Mustafah, and lives in the same village, but he does not know or cannot give a telephone number. We transmit this little information to the people of the Outreach team, hoping that they will be able to find out more. Until that time, since we don't know whether he has had contact with an Ebola case, we do not feel comfortable discharging him.

In my own country, the man would already have had a CT-scan and probably also an MRI of the brain, plus extensive blood work and examination of his cerebral spinal fluid – all on the first day of admission. In any regular hospital, at least the right kind of nursing care would have been started for someone with such a severe level of paralysis, to prevent bedsores and contractures. Here, we can only do our best to keep him alive, and to discharge him as soon as it is safe to the city hospital in Kailahun town, hoping he will get the right kind of care there.

At the end of my shift, I'm tired. We quickly take the Land Cruiser back to the hotel. Dinner, followed by the hour-long weekly meeting with all the expats. It is ten o'clock before we're done. The internet connection is failing again this evening, an extra setback. The wireless internet connection at the hotel is a nice comfort to be able to keep in touch with family, friends and the regular outside world in general, but it has been malfunctioning for the last three evenings. It has never been good enough for Facetime or Skype, like I had planned. Contact with my family is done by frequent brief Whatsapp messages and a daily (password-protected) blog.

# Thursday, November 27

**Andy**
Alimany the midfielder died last night. A young man in the prime of his life robbed of his future.

I am given this news as I enter the EMC, the staff who are finishing their shift know that I spent time with him yesterday and that I would want this information immediately. I thank Mohammed for letting me know and take a walk over to a secluded corner near the store. Here I stand and stare into space. My thoughts and emotions swirl and as often occurs here I find myself with a deep sense of sorrow.

I have to collect myself quickly as this place is about the living and I have blood samples to collect.

Inside High Risk Kenichi and I enter tent C4. Osman is still with us, as is his dad. His dad has deteriorated and his respiratory rate has quickened. He seems distressed and so I give him an injection of morphine to try to cover any pain he may have and to help him settle.

Kenichi focuses his attention on a little boy, of barely a year old, who suffers from cerebral palsy, apart from Ebola, and who is alone in the Confirmed area. He knew the baby's mother and tells me how lovingly she looked after her small son, even when she was very ill herself. The baby's general condition, despite him having cerebral palsy, is testament to her care. Sadly his mother died recently. Kenichi clearly feels a sense of obligation towards the baby now that she is gone. The baby is cared for by some of the ladies in the Confirmed area but they are a little uncomfortable with him due to his cerebral palsy and the fact that this makes him 'different' to the other children. Some of the women call him the 'devil child', which is awful, but people here don't understand things like hypoxic brain damage.

I leave C6 as we approach the end of our permitted time in the High Risk area. Kenichi is sitting on a chair patiently giving the baby milk on a spoon. It is lovely to watch and I stop for a few minutes and take the time to witness this beautiful example of humanity.

**Anna**

Another hot afternoon. The two new expat nurses are on their first afternoon shift with me, after having done their first morning shift yesterday. So today, on my eighth shift, I'm expected to instruct them and help coordinate their activities. Luckily they are both very experienced: Bob from Sweden who has worked on multiple MSF missions before, and Albert from Liberia, who has worked on an MSF Ebola mission before, in Uganda in 2012, so he knows a lot and has only to get up to speed with the way things are set up in Kailahun.

For a large part of the afternoon I'm acting more like a coordinator from the Low Risk zone. Everything is running smoothly. My colleagues are very busy in the High Risk zone with the boy Osman and his father. Unfortunately, both have taken a turn for the worse today. Osman is confused and restless, his father is in a lot of pain and has trouble breathing. We can only try to make them as comfortable as possible, give them medication for the pain and restlessness, and try to give them plenty of fluids. But it is a bad sign, usually when patients reach this stage it does not end well.

I do go into the High Risk zone in PPE three times myself as well. The first time around half past two, just after the handover, to receive an ambulance. I take Albert with me to show him the way our protocol works. The two patients can walk themselves over to triage where we take their temperature and then leave them behind for the triage interview. They are both likely to have Ebola, so they will be admitted. On our way out through the High Risk zone, we administer injections with medication for nausea to two patients. Then we exit quickly because in the early afternoon heat we are already drenched in sweat after only 30 minutes inside.

Just after six o'clock, another unexpected ambulance arrives. Many of the nurses and the other expats have only just left the High Risk zone, so it is my turn again. I go in with Sahr, a local nurse, and sprayer Kellie. The temperature is more bearable now because the sun was setting while we were dressing in PPE. On opening the ambulance we find that it contains two patients. The first is a 42-year old man, who can walk to triage with a little bit of support. He has a fever and a lot of other symptoms, so it is very likely that he has Ebola.

That leaves the second patient: a comatose woman of about 25 years of age lies on the stretcher inside the ambulance. This stretcher is fixed to the vehicle and cannot be pulled out so there is no option but for me to climb into the ambulance, careful not to tear my PPE. Kellie assists in holding our own stretcher against the back of the ambulance while Sahr and I push and pull the woman out, trying to be patient-friendly and yet as safe for ourselves as possible. Next, Sahr and I carry her on the stretcher to triage.

Again, no documentation is provided. The patient has no wristband with her name although she does have a urinary catheter in place, so she must have come from a hospital. She is in quite a deep comatose state, no response to pain, and a fever of 38.4 degrees Celsius. She has a rapid but strong pulse, no clear abrasions, and no obvious loss of blood. That is all we know. It does not seem very useful to leave her in triage in these circumstances, so we decide to carry her into the High Risk zone immediately, and put her on a bed in one of the 'suspect Ebola' tents. Once we get back to the Low Risk zone there will be time to try and find out more information. Sahr and I get hold of the stretcher again and carry her into the High Risk zone, while Kellie opens and closes the gates for us. It is hard work, sweating in the warm PPE, carrying an adult woman on a stretcher, and transferring her from the stretcher to a bed. We can't do much more than put her down, cover her in a blanket and then leave to recover ourselves.

Once I'm back in the Low Risk zone, I wonder how on earth we are going to get more information about her – we do not even have a name. When I discuss it with the team of national nurses, we get lucky: one of the nurses knows a colleague in the hospital that the patient apparently was sent from, a few hours drive away, and he has heard some rumours. I encourage him to phone his friend to find out more. At last we have a name: Sara. It turns out that she gave birth two weeks ago to an apparently healthy baby, but that she started to have convulsions after giving birth. Two days ago, she was admitted to the hospital because the convulsions got worse and worse. At the hospital, they did not know how to help her. Today, they became afraid that she may have Ebola, and the nurses had become reluctant to care for her. So she was put into an ambulance and dropped off on our doorstep. There did not appear to have been any contact with an Ebola patient or an unsafe burial, as far as we can determine.

So what is wrong with her? Ebola seems less likely. More probable is a complication of her pregnancy or delivery, or some other kind of infection, or perhaps epilepsy, or low sugar level. The local hospital in Kailahun town is full (I happen to know this because we wanted to discharge two patients to them today, including Emmanuel, the man with the left-sided paralysis, whom we have now been able to confirm definitely does not have Ebola). After another discussion of the pros and cons, we decide that Sara probably does not have Ebola, but will have to remain with us until we can make sure and find another solution. By this time it is eight o'clock. Just after the handover to the night shift I go back inside for a final time with Bokarie to see Sara again. We start treatment for all the possible treatable causes of her coma. It does not have an immediate effect, and I leave her behind still in a coma.

When I finally get back to the hotel this evening there is a party going on. A birthday party for Tom, the expat who is in charge of human resources, and a farewell party for Bill, our Project Coordinator who is leaving for home tomorrow. A barbecue outside, music, and even banana bread for a birthday cake. I'm very tired, and not really in the mood when I arrive. My mind is still on Sara. While at work in the EMC I'm in professional mode as a doctor and think about her problems in a technical, clinical way. Only now do I allow the full tragedy of the situation to sink in. A previously healthy young woman, who has just given birth, is now in a coma inside our EMC. Probably her family do not even know where she is or whether she is still alive. What are her chances? It sets me to brooding about the inequality in this world. A few fellow expats who have had the day off today and who are enjoying the party cajole me into staying for the food and music. They are right, it is good to take my mind off the day's worries and our limitations for an evening.

# Friday, November 28

**Anna**
Seventh afternoon shift in a row, so another morning off. I missed the visit by the president of Sierra Leone to our EMC. He was flown in by helicopter, with his bodyguards. He was shown around the outside perimeter of the clinic and was informed about the work. It was his second visit to Kailahun this year. From across the fence from the outside he talked with some of the convalescent patients, and he told the employees that he would set up a new committee that would be responsible for the payment of the danger money that has been promised by the government. The fact that this danger money hasn't been paid out is the major reason for the brief strikes that have taken place at several places in Sierra Leone in the past few weeks. The employees of the EMC are working for MSF and receive a salary from MSF, but the government has promised additional danger money for anyone working to stop Ebola.

There are about six or seven patients in the EMC at the moment that are likely to die within the next day or two, with nothing we can do to prevent it. One of those is Osman's father. He has deteriorated greatly, with increasing bleeding and breathing difficulties. Osman is in the bed next to him. The boy seems to be doing a little bit better than yesterday but he is in a dangerous state of health. I sit down next to him for a little while, help him to sit up to eat a little and to drink. I stroke his hair and my gloved hand holds his. He is frightened, and doesn't want us to go. Just imagine, lying in such strange surroundings, people in strange yellow suits coming in, and your father next to you so ill that he can no longer look after you. We have to go, our time in PPE is up, we have to leave the High Risk zone. But I know that everyone has a special place in their heart for Osman, just as for a number of other patients who are alone or need special attention. Everyone tries to visit these patients on each trip into High Risk.

# Saturday, November 29

**Anna**
A day off – not going to the EMC for a day gives us a chance to recharge our batteries. Andy, Bob and I go out for a beautiful long walk, randomly choosing some footpaths from the hotel. Beautiful surroundings, everything grows abundantly here, including banana, mango, coffee, coco, oranges, palm oil, okra, coconut, pineapple. We pass three small villages along narrow footpaths.

Along the way we have brief friendly meetings with the locals. Even in the smallest communities there are posters with information about Ebola. Two men we meet along the way ask us the latest news of the outbreak in their province. As everywhere, small children are excited to see white people "Pumweh!" and come running up. But all of them know about 'no touch' so they do keep their distance. A small boy wisely tells us not to eat monkey meat, because it could give you Ebola. Our walk takes us to the small remote village of Gbojiema where the villagers receive us very kindly. There has been no case of Ebola in their village, but still they feel the effects of the epidemic. There is less work, less business done on the markets and more poverty.

By this time it is noon, time to turn around and head back to the hotel. It is humid and hot, and my T-shirt is covered with sweat markings. I've become more or less used to that in the past two weeks. Back in the base hotel I take a cold shower and relax for a while in my room near the fan. The rest of the afternoon I spend with my laptop in one of the public tukuls of the hotel.

It was a lovely, relaxing day, with the opportunity to see a little bit more of regular life in Sierra Leone. Ebola has its effects outside the EMC as well. This also becomes clear from conversations with the local drivers of the Land Cruiser that takes us to and fro between the hotel and the EMC. That route passes a building which looks like a bar or club. The drivers tell us that indeed it used to be a nightspot, but it has been closed since the Ebola outbreak. Further along the way, after driving out of Kailahun town, we pass a beautiful view across a green valley, mist-covered mountains in the background. This is the border area. The mountains we see in the distance are a few kilometres away in Guinea; and a car can take you to Liberia, in the other direction, within half an hour. A river runs through the bottom of the valley, flanked by sandy banks. On those banks, people from Guinea, Sierra Leone and Liberia used to gather – it is a favourite spot to spend Christmas together. All that has ended since the advent of Ebola as the borders have been closed and it is forbidden to gather in large groups. Christmas will be very different this year.

Francis, one of the other drivers, tells us about his brothers and sisters, who all live in Monrovia in Liberia. He has not seen them or spoken to them in the last few months. He has tried calling them on their mobile, but there is no answer. He hopes that they have just changed their phone number and forgot to inform him. As soon as the outbreak is over he wants to travel to Monrovia to look for them. Many people here are separated from relatives in Guinea, Liberia or in remote areas of Sierra Leone because of Ebola.

It was obvious on our walk today that the extensive education about Ebola in the past months has had a good effect in Kailahun. In the beginning, people were mostly scared and panicking. When MSF leased the land to build the EMC just outside Kailahun town the first response was to protest. But a lot of education and good leadership changed that into support. Francis, who has worked here from the start, tells us that the stretch of land was leased on a Sunday and within one week 100 to 200 local workers helped to clear the land of all the trees and vegetation and to build the EMC out of nothing, so that the first patients could be admitted within two weeks. MSF is very much appreciated here both for the work they do for Ebola patients and as an employer. This is an area where work has always been scarce, and has become more so in the past six months. Francis explains that the part of the compound across the road from the EMC, with the carpentry workshop, National Staff clinic etc was nearly all built by volunteers from the community. They wanted to do their bit to help in the epidemic, and they also wanted to increase their chances of paid work with MSF.

In the last few weeks, the Ebola outbreak in the province of Kailahun has greatly diminished. We only get a handful of new patients every week from the direct surroundings. Most patients now come from far away. The western and northern areas of the country, where the epidemic is much more active at the moment, have a great shortage of active EMCs, despite many good intentions. So far, people in Kailahun accept that their area will host sick people from other districts. No one has suggested we refuse patients from far away, no cries of, "Stay in your own district, don't bring Ebola back here!" I wonder whether it would be the same in any Western country.

## Andy

Three thousand miles away, back in Harrogate UK, it is Burlesque Without Borders 8 tonight. This event is part of the walka2b project that I have been running for the last five years with the support of an amazing group of friends. In 2009 I decided that I wanted to keep my connection with MSF in between missions. Raising money to support their work seemed the obvious way to accomplish this. The original focus of the project was a long distance walk from Amsterdam to Barcelona. This three and a half month, 2,000 mile walk took in the five European headquarters of MSF in Amsterdam, Brussels, Paris, Geneva and Barcelona. The walk was the focus but many events sprung up as part of the on-going fundraising effort, the most notable being Burlesque Without Borders. BWB is the brainchild of my friend Lily la Belle and has already raised over £8000. The show is a wonderful blend of dance, music, magic and lovely people taking their clothes off. The appeal would seem obvious!

I am sad to be missing the night but I am pleased that Tracey is going with her friends from the Armed Forces Fitness group. It is good to know that she has such good friends to keep her company. Her best pal

Darren is especially kind and looks out for her knowing that this is a tough time.

At seven o'clock I sit on my bed refreshing the painfully slow internet connection to Facebook. With the 'patience of Job' I am able to see some photos from the show via emails. The photos take so long to download it hurts! Despite the slow connection it is heartening to feel like I am part of the night even when I am so far away. Lily even reads out a message from me thanking everyone in the 200 strong audience for coming and once again asks them to give their money to MSF. By midnight over £1,000 is raised.

# Sunday, November 30

**Anna**
Morning shift. Bad news about little Osman and his father; the father died yesterday morning, Osman is very sad and is deteriorating day by day. He seems to be suffering from kidney failure, although we don't have the tests available to confirm it. It wouldn't make any difference though because we can't treat him for it. We can only relieve his suffering.

I'm doing the rounds in the 'probable Ebola' tents today, together with CHO Amara and nurse Sheku. These tents are extra full today because yesterday around half past six in the evening, two full ambulances arrived from Freetown, more than 400km away. The 11 patients from those two vehicles are very ill. One of them did not survive the trip and was 'dead on arrival'. Pain, vomiting, diarrhoea everywhere – two patients have the hiccups, one of the bad signs in Ebola. We try to see and talk to everyone to prescribe medication and to decide whether they should get a fluid infusion.

This takes us to the bed of the morbidly ill man that I described at the start of this book, whose name is unknown to us. The other patients on this round include a teenage brother and sister, a number of young adults in their twenties and ten-year-old Musa. The boy Musa has arrived alone, without any family. He lives in a small village near Freetown and has visited the traditional funeral of his uncle. His parents have probably died from Ebola and we know that his grandmother is also ill. Clearly, Ebola education has not yet reached all villages and communities in other parts of Sierra Leone.

Squatting down next to Musa's bed to take his temperature, I take hold of his hand to put him at his ease. He understands and speaks English quite well. I introduce myself. My name, Anna, is also written on my forehead in big red letters, on the white hood. This evokes a touching response from the boy: he squeezes my hand and tells me that his mother is also called Anna. How do you respond to that?

There is so much to do that Amara and I do not succeed in seeing all the patients we are supposed to. When we have seen and tended to 12 patients we get a shouted warning from across the fence: we have been inside the High Risk in PPE for 70 minutes already, that's past the limit. Quick calculation: that means less than six minutes per very ill patient – including assessment, care and giving medication. We quickly let the last two patients know that someone will come to see them as soon as possible. We still have to call our findings on the patients across the fence to the medical clerk on duty. We are drenched in sweat by the time we get undressed.

Let me not forget the one positive highlight of this morning's rounds. A young woman is seated on a chair outside one of the tents in the "suspected Ebola" area, cleanly washed and dressed, eating biscuits. She still has a kind of dazed look in her eyes, but she understands what we say to her. I don't recognise her but this is Sara, the young woman who was brought in in a coma a few days ago! Her Ebola tests have remained negative, and despite the dreadful circumstances she has survived, and has woken up from her coma. We still don't know the cause. Possibly in the hospital she was just given too many sedatives for her convulsions. This afternoon she can leave our EMC. Hopefully she will recover fully, and will be able to go home soon to her newborn baby.

Before my morning shift is over, the man without a name who was so ill is found dead in his bed.

## Andy

This afternoon I enter High Risk with Kenichi. We intend to focus on tent C4. The young boy Osman, is outside the tent on a mat as his temperature is elevated. After giving him rectal paracetamol to help reduce his fever my colleagues had taken him outside where there is some air movement. He is so poorly, hardly responsive. I will be surprised if he survives the day. He does at least appear comfortable at present.

Once we are reassured of Osman's immediate safety we move on to carry out a rapid assessment of the patients inside the tent and to perform the tasks we pre-planned. Intravenous fluids and pain relief are the main focus of this round. Intravenous fluid administration has started again following the incident when the fluid bag fell to the floor and backfilled with blood. The decision was made that we can restart but we cannot leave drips running, we have to push in as much fluid as we can in the one hour we are present and then take the drip down.

I am struggling with the heat today, it is hot, very hot. Temperatures up to 46 degrees Celsius have been measured inside the protective equipment that we are wearing and right now I'm feeling every degree. Beads of sweat collect in my goggles and I have a constant awareness of the mask over my mouth and nose, which makes breathing a conscious effort.

Kenichi and I manage to put in cannulas in three patients and give a litre of fluids to each of them. We also set up a rapid drip on a very dehydrated lady. The team has done a great job with her today, she has had three litres in about four hours and by the end of it she is looking loads better. Her sunken eyes have filled out, her mouth is less dry and she is a lot more alert.

At seven o'clock in the evening, Bob, our Swedish nurse, approaches me in the Low Risk area and says, "The very sick boy in C4, Osman, could do with a last look before we finish. He is making some gurgling sounds and I'm worried about leaving him on the mat." Bob is right to be concerned, the sounds could indicate that Osman is not clearing his airway properly. I decide to go back into the High Risk area once more to assess him before I finish my day at the EMC. I find Osman still on the mat outside the tent. His airway and breathing seem safe but it is getting cold now that the sun has gone down. Amara, my National Staff colleague, and I pick him up and move him into the tent and onto his bed. We then turn him to his side and support him with blankets. He responds little to our intervention but by the time we are ready to leave he looks comfortable. I stroke his head and whisper some reassurance that is as much for me as it is for him and then I leave him for the night.

I have sweated and sweated today. I changed my scrubs three times. My socks and pants were wet with perspiration but I couldn't change them. I drank around five litres to compensate and will consume a further 500ml before bed. It is physically draining work that leaves my skin looking like I have been in the bath too long when I take off my double layer gloves. I take the wet socks off and come home in just the shoes tonight.

By half past ten I am in bed and ready for sleep. It has been a tough day but we have done some good.

*New Ebola hospitals*

In September and October 2014 MSF spoke out that the help given to West Africa and the Ebola epidemic was insufficient. At that time most new cases of Ebola in Sierra Leone occurred in Freetown and the northern provinces of the country. However, the only significant EMC's in the country were the two MSF centres in Bo (in the middle of the country) and Kailahun (in the east), and an EMC of the International Red Cross in Kenema, which is located between Bo and Kailahun.

The ambulances that arrived in our Kailahun EMC from Freetown or Tonkolili had completed a hellish trip. The patients took the same road that we did on our arrival, a distance of more than 400 km. The same distance as that from Nijmegen in The Netherlands to Paris in France or from London to Newcastle upon Tyne in the UK, the final stretch of the journey being on a rough dirt road. Imagine falling ill in Nijmegen, nauseated, suffering from diarrhoea and in pain and hearing that you will be taken to Paris in a packed Land Cruiser without stops along the way and the last two hours will be along a bumpy soil road, while your relatives, staying behind in Nijmegen will not be able to visit you.

The UK Government had instructed the British army to build an Ebola hospital in the west of Sierra Leone in October, but they had chosen to build a semi-permanent building of bricks and mortar. This took 3 months to build, and after that, personnel still needed to be hired and trained. Three months may sound like a short time to build a hospital, but when a deadly epidemic is ravaging the country it is much too long.

While the response of other aid organisations lagged behind, MSF decided by mid November to build two new tent EMC's, one in Freetown and one in the northern district of Magburaka. Within three weeks those EMC's were ready, personnel had been hired, training started and the first patients could be admitted.

Looking back, Kailahun received the last ambulances from far away on November 30. From December 1 the expected opening of new EMC's in the west was imminent and patients in the holding centres in the west and north of the country were kept there to wait for those new centres. From that day onwards, our work in Kailahun changed for the better, slowly (and in the beginning hardly perceptibly), as patient numbers began to fall.

# Monday, December 1

**Andy**

It is half past six and I am in High Risk taking the morning blood samples. Anna's goggles fogged a few minutes ago and she had to leave the High Risk zone. I manage to take the remaining samples but need three attempts on one poor man. I apologise profusely via Susan, my National Staff colleague. It is clear that he doesn't mind in the slightest and expresses his gratitude for the care he is receiving, which is very touching.

Susan translates the man's next comments for me, "You are very nice. In the government holding centre the staff kicked food towards us as they were too scared to come near." I don't know what to say to this so I say nothing.

Poor Osman is still with us, now alone after the death of his father. He clings to his young life. We treat his symptoms and monitor for any sign that he is uncomfortable. We keep him clean and turn him for pressure area care and comfort.

I enter High Risk again around half past twelve along with Sarah from the National Staff and Albert, a Liberian nurse who has significant experience in Ebola. We are soon in PPE and head for the Confirmed area to visit a little girl in C4 – Kadiatu. She is two years old and came to the EMC in an ambulance with her grandfather. Her grandfather was tested but was found to be negative for Ebola so he was discharged and she is alone. Kadiatu is clearly dehydrated and listless. I discuss her case with Albert. We decide that we should set up a drip to give the little girl both fluid and some glucose. It is possible that her drowsiness is due to a low blood sugar level. Soon after the fluids have infused she starts to show signs of improvement. The signs are quite subtle; she simply seems a little more alert. Both Albert and I feel satisfied with our work. I think we are all able to empathise with the plight of this little child who has no one to sit with her and to reassure her except for the staff in full PPE.

Opposite Kadiatu is a lady who in truth I know little about. I can however see that she is very sick. She looks so sad. I go to her and make a quick assessment with Sarah. The lady, Fatmata, has pain in her joints and a sore throat. Her temperature is elevated and she looks dehydrated. She already has a cannula in her arm and after my assessment I give her a rapid 500ml of intravenous fluid. We still encourage her to try a drink and she manages to take a small volume of ORS plus some pain relief. The final thing I give her is a hug, easily forgotten but vital.

After I hand over to the afternoon shift, a group of us take a walk to the nearby Moa River. The river is only about 20 minutes from the EMC and marks the Sierra Leone – Guinea border. In my mind rivers always evoke a feeling of freedom. As we chat among ourselves, a group of children and a woman approach the riverbank. The children play in the water and the lady starts to wash clothes. Once again, normality coexists with the grossly abnormal situation of Ebola.

For a few minutes it is almost possible to forget that we are 20 minutes walk away from the EMC and 15 minutes from the vast cemetery.

**Anna**

I've been on morning shift today but I see the EMC again this evening. After dinner, when all the expats have returned to the hotel, there is a message from the EMC. The lights have gone out in one of the patients' tents. This is a safety hazard for staff who need to enter High Risk at night for their rounds. Steve, the Canadian logistician who deals with such things at the centre, will go back to try to fix the problem. I volunteer to accompany him back to the EMC to assist.

We go into the Low Risk area, in the familiar green scrubs and white boots, with a large box of tools, wiring and lamps from the workshop across the road. Steve dresses in PPE, with someone from the WatSan team as his buddy, and enters High Risk. I stay behind on the Low Risk side with the box of gear, at the fence near to the tent that is in darkness. It doesn't take long before I see the shadows of Steve and his buddy inside the tent, working by torchlight. Within a few seconds the light comes on. Steve leaves the tent and walks up to me. All he has done is put a plug in an electrical outlet, and the light worked again. He suspects one of the patients has just pulled out the plug to get better sleep. It can't be very comfortable to be lying in a brightly lit tent all night, especially when you're not feeling well.

But while we are chatting across the fence, suddenly something happens. Did a light behind me just go dark, a second ago, or did we imagine it? Before we can decide what really happened, all the lights go out. The whole EMC, High Risk zone, Low Risk zone, everywhere, covered in darkness. Not good. There are people in PPE in the High Risk zone, who are now in pitch black. Steve and his buddy are the only ones carrying torches.

At first I am amazed that there is no panic or unrest either among patients or staff. But then I realise that in Kailahun a fixed source of electricity is unknown. Some rich families or public buildings possess a generator that is turned on at night but that is still a luxury and it is not uncommon for such generators to fail now and then. The sun-powered streetlights along the main street in Kailahun town were only installed a year ago. So the absence of light is very normal here. Torches are calmly distributed. The people in the High Risk zone all move towards the undressing tents, where they undress by the light of multiple torches.

Steve and his buddy decide to remain inside for now. Steve gives me instructions about the location of the generator in the area across the road from the EMC, and how I can try to get it going again. I manage to find the generator hut. It is dark and filled with a balmy heat. I use my torch to light the operating panel of the generator and try to remember the right order to push the buttons, according to Steve's instructions. I try to ignore the hundreds of insects attracted by my torch. All my efforts are in vain. I push the buttons but nothing happens. I give up. This problem needs an expert. Back in the EMC, Steve and his buddy are still waiting in PPE, in the dark. Steve needs to go and fix the generator himself, if possible. Carefully, he and his buddy are helped to undress safely in the dark undressing tents, lit by torchlight.

For me, the next hour or so involves a lot of waiting around while Steve and a local handyman who happened to be on duty tonight try to get the generator going. It has overheated and is now apparently unable to cope with lighting up the whole EMC. They have to find a way to light a number of essential areas, at least one of the dressing tents and one undressing tent. The lighting in other areas, such as most of the Low Risk zone, will have to wait until tomorrow. With the help of some strategically placed extension cords we finally manage to get enough light for the night shift to get by. The National Staff are fine with that – like I mentioned, they are used to dealing with darkness. At last, Steve and I can take the car back to the hotel, where we arrive around 11 pm. I'm glad I'm not on morning shift tomorrow.

# Tuesday, December 2

**Andy**

Once again I sit opposite a patient for blood sampling. This time I have to make a distinct effort to clear my mind. I have just had an argument with Laura. While setting up for my previous sample she was shouting requests to me over the fence from Low Risk, "Can you check tent S1 for syringes," "Can you check patient 1470's temperature?" I told her to shut up, as this is no time for distractions. She doesn't take blood or cannulate and so doesn't run the risk. She is seemingly unaware of the danger of distracting those that do.

In truth Laura has caused a few problems in the team since we arrived from Holland. Eliseo is by far the best at being pissed off with her. He has an extremely expressive face and has mastered the gestures that make Italian footballers famous the world over! She repeatedly fails to adhere to the instructions we were given in Amsterdam regarding not changing the system in the EMC. Worse, she invariably goes over the time limit inside High Risk. Whenever I am coordinating I have to bloody well tell her that she is over the hour. Only yesterday she overstayed her time in C4. By the time she left High Risk (with her National Staff partner whom she is supposed to look after), it was 1 hour and 30 minutes. I was furious and asked the Medical Team Leader to speak to her. As expats we are responsible for our National Staff colleagues. We cannot put them in a position where they feel obliged to stay in High Risk just because the expat happens to be 'fine'. It is selfish, dangerous and in my opinion abusive.

Once I have completed the blood sampling, I call into C4 to see Osman before I leave High Risk. The poor lad is still alive but is puffed up with what I suspect is kidney failure. His eyes are nearly closed due to the swelling.

A lady in her 40s called Amie is next to him but as I look at her I can see right away that she has died. I confirm her death. Osman is too sick to comprehend all of this; at least I hope he is. As I leave High Risk I think about this lady and also Fatmata, the lady I hugged yesterday. She too died overnight.

I leave the EMC feeling quite low today, in truth the death and the suffering of the patients plays on my mind. I often wake up in the early hours dreaming about them. I mull this over in the Land Cruiser back to base. I decide that it's probably normal in the circumstances. That said I feel the need to lay off some of my anger and frustration and who better to aim it at than my MP! It is sheer fortune that MSF chose today to issue a further communication, which fires me up.

International Ebola response slow and piecemeal, risks becoming a 'double failure' says MSF
LONDON, 2 December 2014 –

*The international response to Ebola in West Africa has so far been patchy and slow, and has left local people, national governments and non-governmental organisations (NGOs) to do most of the practical, hands-on work. The international medical humanitarian organisation Doctors Without Borders/Médecins Sans Frontières (MSF) warned today that the international community must not fail twice with a response that is slow in the first instance and ill-adapted later on.*

*Three months after MSF called for states with biological-disaster response capacity to urgently dispatch human and material resources to West Africa, all three of the worst-hit countries have received some assistance from the international community. But foreign governments have focused primarily on financing or building Ebola case management structures, leaving staffing them up to national authorities, local healthcare staff and NGOs which do not have the expertise required to do so. The national authorities in the affected countries have taken the lead on the response with the means available to them.*

*"Training NGOs and local healthcare workers to safely operate case management facilities takes weeks. Though MSF and other organisations have been offering training, this bottleneck has created huge delays," says Dr Joanne Liu, MSF's International President. "It is extremely disappointing that states with biological-disaster response capacities have chosen not to deploy them. How is it that the international community has left the response to Ebola – now a transnational threat – up to doctors, nurses and charity workers?"*

*Across the region, there are still not adequate facilities for isolating and diagnosing patients where they are needed. In rural areas of Liberia where there are active chains of transmission, for example, there are no transport facilities for laboratory samples. In Sierra Leone, scores of people calling in to the national Ebola hotline to report a suspected case are told to isolate the person at home.*

> *Meanwhile, other elements that are essential to an Ebola response – such as awareness-raising and community acceptance, safe burials, contact tracing, alert and surveillance – are still lacking in parts of West Africa. In Guinea, for example, where the epidemic continues to spread, awareness raising and sensitisation remains very weak – especially for an intervention that began eight months ago. But some international actors seem unable to adapt quickly enough to a fluid situation and shift their focus to other activities as required. "Controlling an Ebola outbreak goes beyond isolation and patient care. Wherever there are new cases the full package of activities must be in place. Everyone involved in the response must take a flexible approach and allocate resources to the most pressing needs at any given time and place across the region," says Dr Liu. "People are still dying horrible deaths in an outbreak that has already killed thousands. We can't let our guard down and allow this to become a 'double failure': a response that is slow to begin with, and then is ill-adapted in the end."*

With this in mind, I take a seat at my laptop and compose a heartfelt email to Andrew Jones the Member of Parliament for Harrogate:

*Dear Mr Jones,*

*I am currently in my third week in MSF's Kailahun Ebola Management Centre in Eastern Sierra Leone. I know that you will be keeping up to date with events in West Africa as you sent me a very positive reply to my original email.*

*Yesterday however MSF issued a press release that heavily criticises the "global community" for their failure to deploy bio response units (as I too mentioned in my original email). I know that the British Army have been active in construction and UKMed are supporting care for medical staff who are infected. This however does not solve the problems mentioned in paragraph 2 of the MSF release.*

*Without properly trained staff these centres can become overwhelmed and do more harm than good. Some of the holding centres in Sierra Leone are thought of as concentration camps by the patients that have come to our EMC.*

*This is a dreadful situation Mr Jones, I look into the eyes of people who are dying every day and it hurts.*

I then add the story of Alimany, closing with:

*Alimany the midfielder died last night. A young man in the prime of his life robbed of his future.*

*People are travelling hundreds of miles across this country to get to functioning EMCs.*

*Ambulances with ten people in can arrive here and sometimes we open doors to find one or two people have died en route. The lack of functioning centres is killing people, MSF can do a lot, it can't do it all. This 'global community' needs to put people with knowledge and skills into Sierra Leone and the region as a whole NOW. Concrete structures and promises aren't enough.*

*Please could I ask you to pass this message to the Minister responsible and to advocate for a commitment to deploying human beings with skills and knowledge to help the general population?*

*It's already too late for many.*

*Thank you for reading my long message and I look forward to your reply.*

*Kind regards*

*Andy Dennis*
*MSF Field Nurse / Staff Nurse Harrogate District Hospital*

This was definitely therapeutic for me and despite the day's tragic events I think I may sleep better tonight.

**Anna**
Just two weeks on the job, and I'm being trained to take on extra responsibilities. Russ, the experienced Canadian MSF doctor, has worked as so-called 'clinical focal point' (CFP) since about a week before we arrived, and he is about to leave for home in a few days. I have been asked to take over the job of CFP once he leaves.

The CFP is the medical expat in the EMC responsible for medical care and decisions on an individual patient level (in contrast to the Medical Manager, who manages the EMC medical National Staff, and the Medical Team Leader who is the head of all medical activities in the project). Straightforward medical decisions around diagnosis or care are taken immediately at the bedside, of course. More complicated matters are discussed within the team of expat doctors and nurses and the CHO on duty. If a decision has to be made, the CFP has the final word. Responsibilities include the interpretation of the Ebola test results (Does the patient have Ebola or not? Is he cured or not? Is he ready for discharge?), the triage decisions about new patients, and decisions about treatment, for example, whether a patient should be given intravenous fluids.

The CFP works an 'in-between' shift starting at ten o'clock in the morning, until around six in the afternoon. This means an overlap of a few hours with the morning shift as well as the afternoon shift, so that you are present for any discussions. Of course the regular work continues, going into the High Risk Zone to tend to patients, etc. I think it will be a good challenge. Out of interest I had already been paying extra attention to the interpretation of the test results in the past two weeks. This will now stand me in good stead.

It is a bit weird to think that after two or three weeks here I am already a veteran. The two expat doctors and one nurse who have been here longer than Andy and I will be leaving for home by the end of this week. However, in such intense settings, the learning curve is steep.

In the early afternoon heat I enter the High Risk zone in PPE, this time for an intravenous (IV) fluid round. My focus this time is three patients in tent C4, Michael, Amie and Kadiatu. Amie, a woman of my own age, arrived two days ago in one of the ambulances from Freetown, very ill and hardly responding. She has recovered a little already. I put down my equipment on a chair nearby, which I have first cleaned, and squat down next to her bed. Her intravenous cannula still looks OK. I carefully connect a new litre bag of fluid, hanging it from one of the tent poles above her, and open it up. The fluid runs in very nicely. Next, it's Michael's turn. He is a 36-year old man who has been with us for a few days now. It is hard to get through to him, somehow. He keeps very quiet, and hardly responds to our questions or conversation, although he is clearly recovering. He seems to be staring at the tent wall most of the time. He gives the impression that he has been traumatised by something – perhaps in the long civil war that ended ten years ago – or has some other psychiatric illness. I have to be persistent in my request that he turns on his back so I can reach the arm with the IV cannula, but finally he allows me to get to it and I start his IV fluid going as well. He immediately moves back on his side, but luckily this doesn't block his cannula and the fluid runs in as fast as before. The last patient is little Kadiatu, the two-year old girl. The poor child is very ill but we hope the IV fluids will give her a chance to recover.

After I have all three IV fluid bags going, I turn my attention to other tasks in the same tent. A cup of ORS for Amie and two of the other women in the tent, changing Kadiatu's diapers, arranging for some clean clothes for one of the other patients. I also give Kadiatu some medication in her IV drip. When I'm nearing the end of my hour in PPE, it is time to push through the remains of the IV fluid, uncouple the IV fluid bags and inject the cannula with some saline to make sure it won't clog up. Finally I bandage it up carefully, so that the patient is less likely to remove it as soon as I am away.

At the end of the hour I emerge from the PPE, wet through again from sweat – my scrubs are drenched, the trousers as well as the shirt. It is always most extreme in the middle of the day. First thing to do is to rehydrate myself with water and ORS. It is now a standing joke to suggest that we also put in an IV cannula for each other and run in a bag of fluid each time we come out of PPE.

On my return to the hotel I find a present from my brother Huib in the email. He has sent me an iTunes music album, a Donizetti opera with Maria Callas in the title role. Beautiful music to divert my thoughts from Ebola and to reconnect with my family far away.

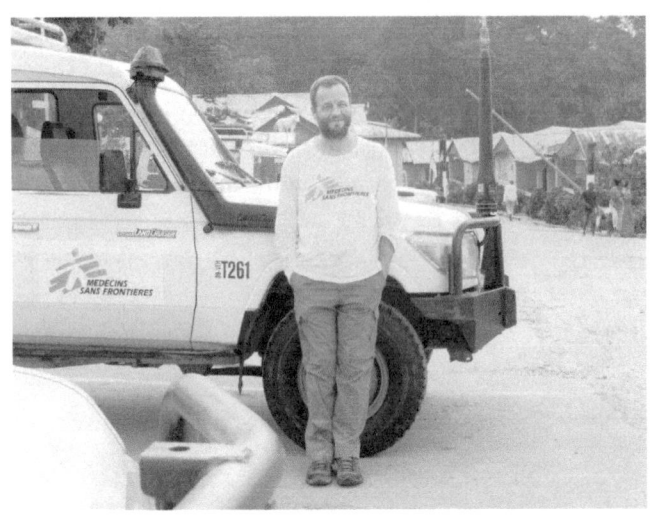

*Andy leaning on one of the MSF Land Cruisers at the base hotel compound. (Photo by Elfriede Thiessens).*

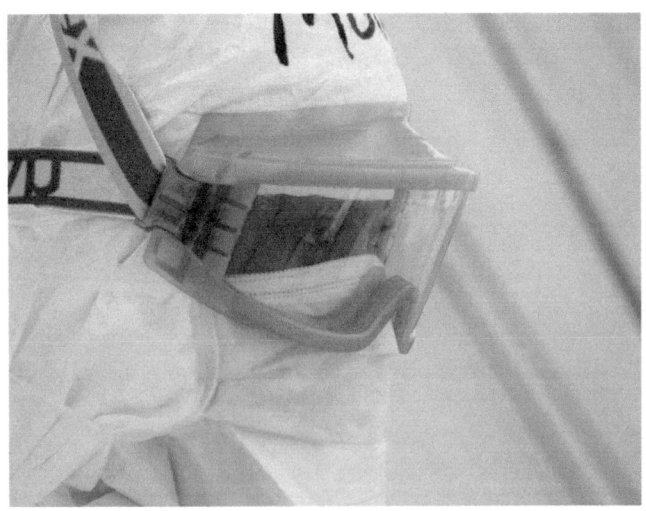

*National Staff nurse in PPE.*

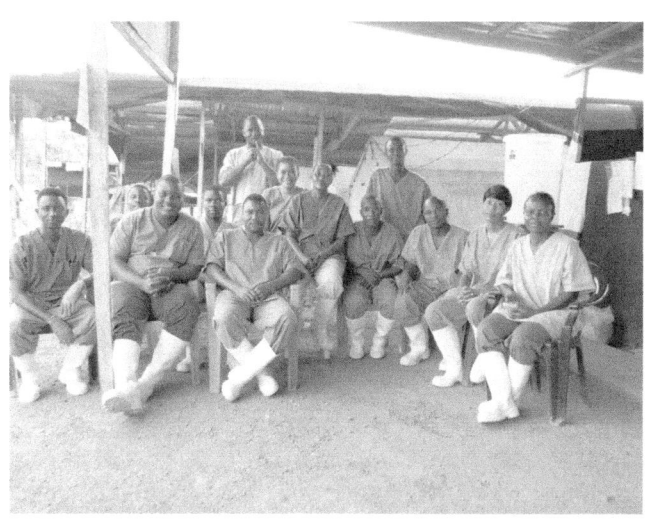

*One of the teams of National Staff nurses and nursing aides in front of the medical tent in the Low Risk area of the EMC.*

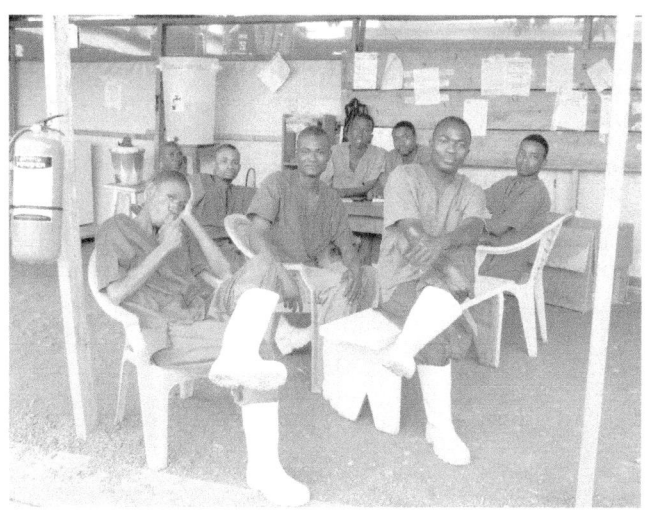

*A group of National Staff members of the Wat-San team, taking a break in their hut in the Low Risk area of the EMC.*

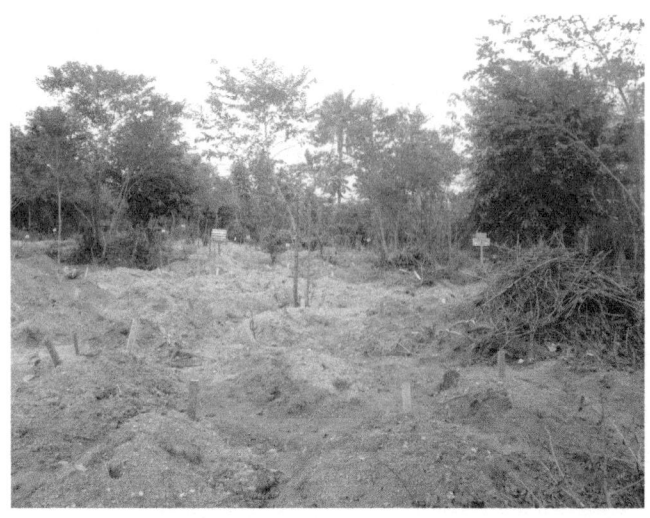

*View of part of the graveyard, a few minutes walk from the EMC in Kailahun. The stake of the grave in the foreground only reads 'DOA' – 'Dead on arrival', with a date.*

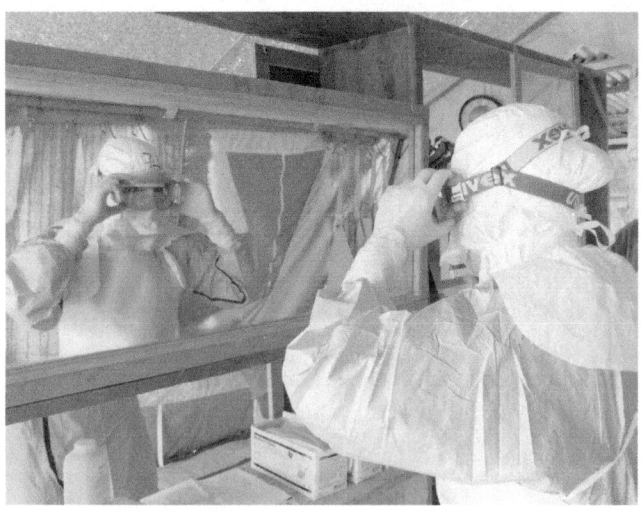

*Crucial last stage of dressing in PPE inside the dressing tent: checking that the safety goggles cover every last bit of skin.*

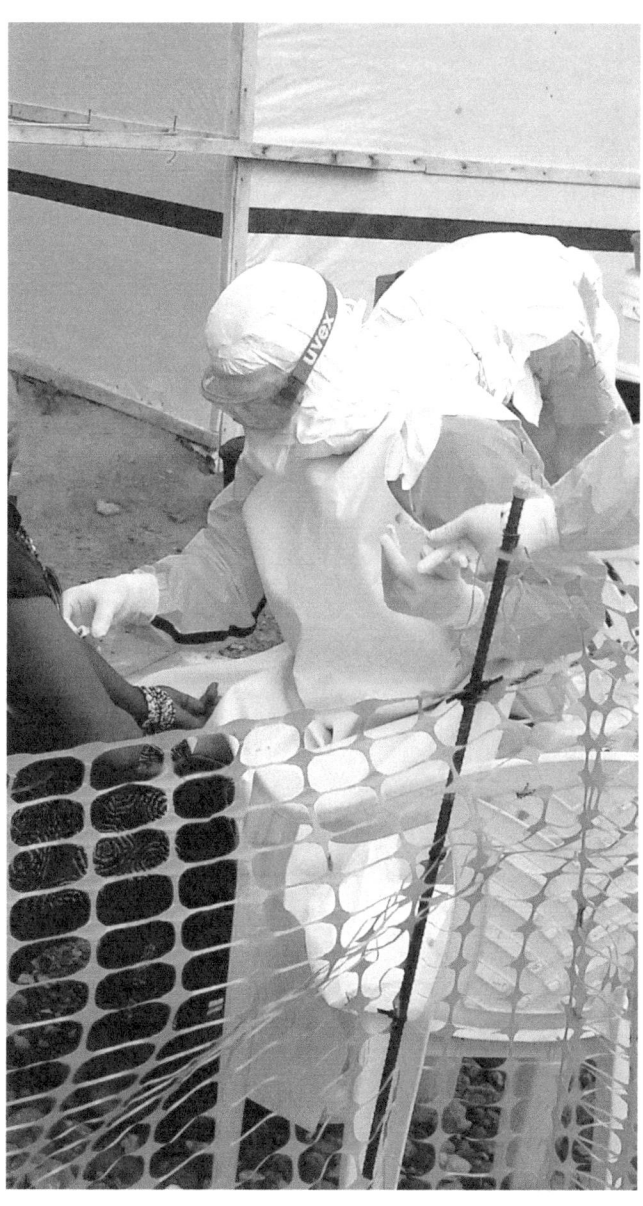

*Andy collecting a blood sample from a convalescing Ebola patient. (Photo by Yves –lyre Marcellus).*

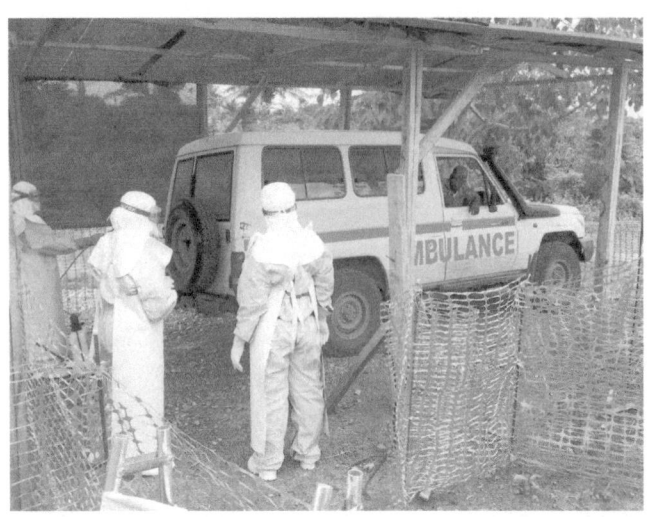

*Arrival of an ambulance at the EMC. The back doors are sprayed with chlorine.*

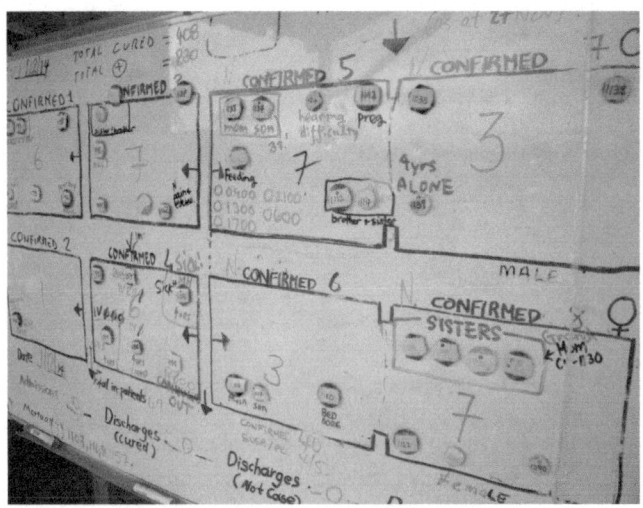

*Part of the whiteboard in the medical tent on which we kept track of the patients in the EMC.*

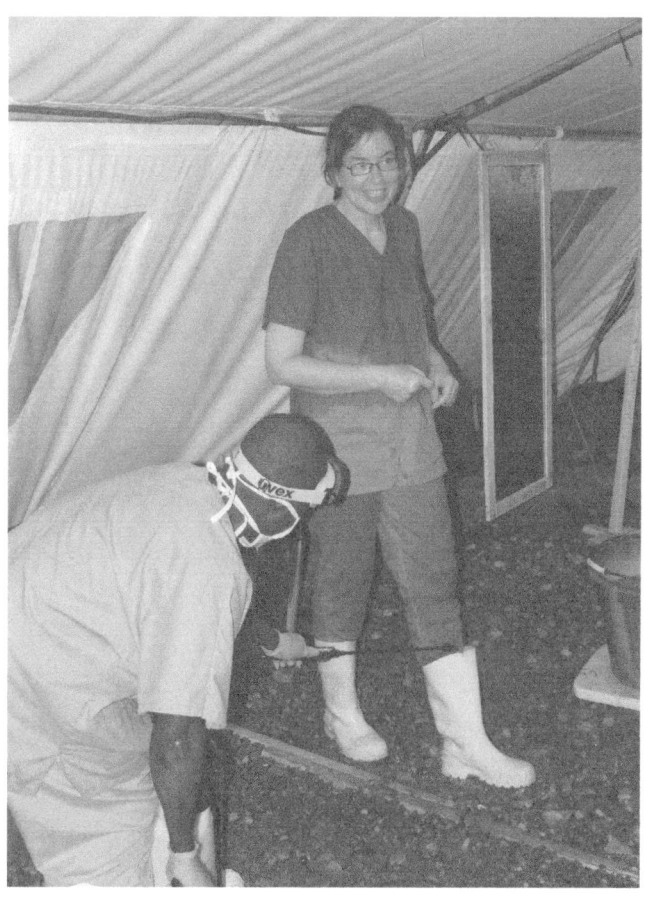

*Anna in the undressing tent, wet from sweat after emerging from an hour in PPE.*

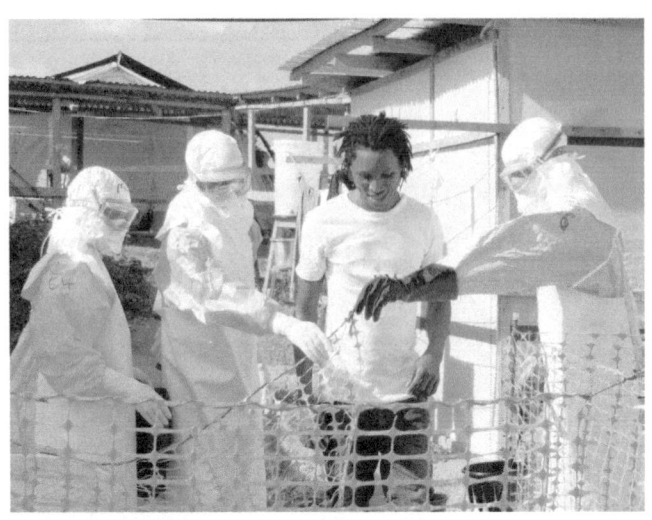

*The moment that Patrik exits the High Risk area of the EMC, upon being declared cured of Ebola (see December 7)*

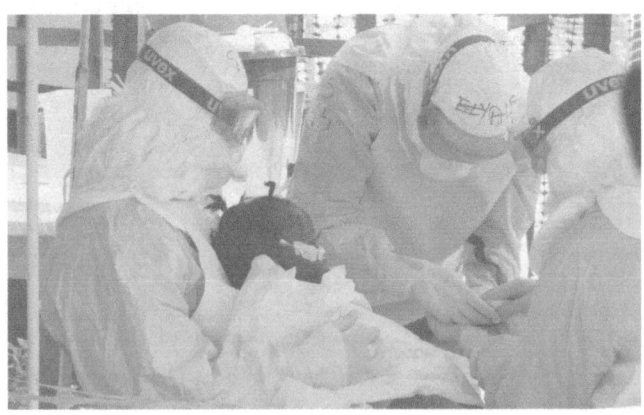

*Bandaging little Kadiatu's hands to prevent her from removing the naso-gastric tube (see December 11)*

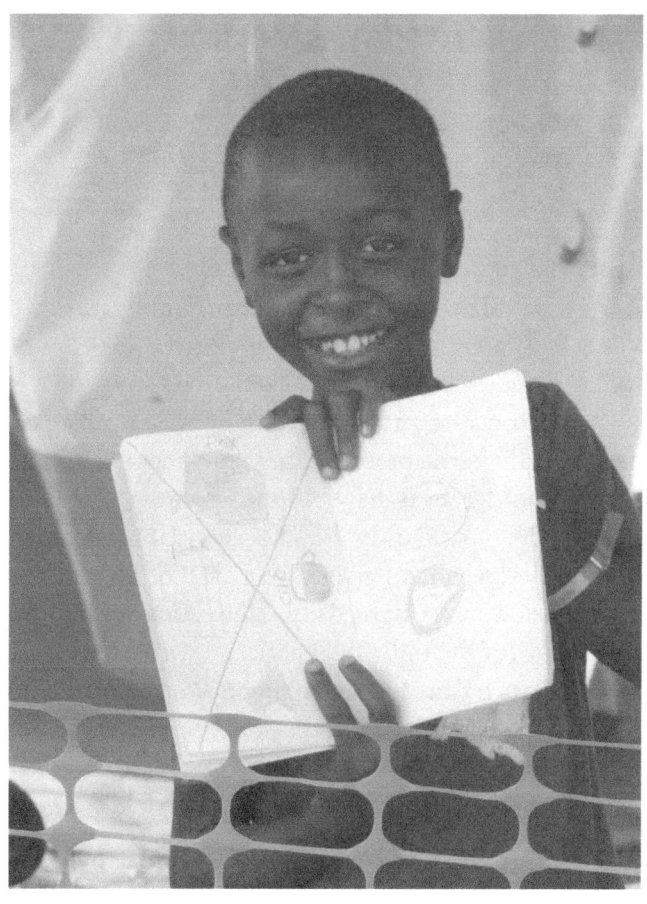

*Musa showing off his drawings in the Convalescent area (see December 11)*

# Wednesday, December 3

**Anna**

A very hot day, even for Kailahun. Going into the High Risk area in PPE is a very extreme experience today. I emerge completely soaked each time.

The number of patients in our EMC has dropped dramatically in the past few days, now that the ambulances from far away have stopped coming. We have gone from 77 patients in the EMC and 10 new admissions each day when I arrived to a total of 36 patients and 1-3 new admissions daily. This means we can do a lot more for the individual patients; we literally have twice as much time for each patient. We have the time to give each patient a good check up. We are able safely to give more patients IV fluids. We can sit down with a patient and just have an encouraging, friendly little chat once in a while.

Andy and I go into the High Risk zone together for an IV round. Kadiatu, the two-year-old girl, needs a new IV cannula. I gently hold her down, while Andy tries to find access. Fortunately, he succeeds. She is still very ill, and is hardly able to drink, let alone take her medication.

Little Osman has surprised everyone today. He has woken up from his comatose state. He is drinking much better and even eating a little. It is tragic to hear him shout for his father. He seems to have forgotten that his father is dead and, for the moment, we hesitate to tell him again. He is still very weak and is not out of danger yet. If he loses hope, he will certainly not survive. Musa, the ten-year-old boy whose mother's name was Anna too, is doing a lot better. Eliseo has given him an empty notebook and some colouring pencils and he makes beautiful drawings.

Later that afternoon I sit in front of the medical tent completing some patient notes, when Laura, the American doctor, walks by towards a group of National Staff nurses sitting a few metres away.

"I want to go in for an IV round. Who will go with me?" she asks the group. They look reluctant. One of the nurses quickly dives into the medical tent, seemingly to perform a chore; another walks away towards the latrines. Usually, we can always find someone to volunteer to help. However, Laura's tendency to stay inside High Risk over the maximum time allowed is well known. She is very passionate about providing care for the patients, and has trouble accepting our limitations here. The National Staff really don't like going inside High Risk with her anymore.

Before things get embarrassing, I get up and offer to go in with her. I think I will have no trouble saying 'no' if she asks me to stay in longer than an hour. This way, I can keep an eye on her to make sure she complies with safety protocols. Joined by a hygienist from the WatSan team, we go to tent C4 to give some IV fluids. Things start off OK, but before long Laura tells me, "You can handle this tent, right? I want to go to C3, and give the young man there some IV fluids as well." And before I can answer she walks away.

I'm kept busy in C4, helped by the hygienist, for the remainder of the hour, finishing the IV drips just in time. At the end of our hour both the hygienist and I are tired, hot and ready to go. Laura has not appeared again. I walk over to tent C3, where she is still busy with her patient.

"Let's go, Laura, we've been inside for an hour," I tell her.

"Just give me a few minutes," she replies, with annoyance in her voice, "This IV is not done yet."

"No Laura, we can't stay. I'm hot, we have to leave."

"No, no, you go. I'm OK, I just want to finish this IV fluid bag."

"Laura, you know I can't leave you behind on your own. Let me help you finish this off, and then we'll go." I try to remain calm, but Laura is clearly not listening to reason. Sweating and tired in PPE is not the best condition for a rational discussion.

Meanwhile, by coincidence, or perhaps by design, Jacques has walked up to the tent. He is the expat from Haiti in charge of water and sanitation, and he is in High Risk with a team of hygienists for a cleaning round. He has been in Kailahun for several weeks longer than Laura and I.

Jacques quickly assesses the situation. "Anna, you go out and undress, I will stay with Laura and get her to leave as well."

Thankfully, I grab the opportunity to leave.

Later, when he is back in the Low Risk area, Jacques tells me how Laura committed another serious breach of the safety protocol. At Jacques' insistence, she finally finished the IV infusion in the patient. When she disconnected the infusion set from the cannula, it leaked some blood before she could cap it and she ended up with blood on her gloved hands. This happens to all of us sometimes. However she then proceeded to rummage about in a storage box inside the tent, with her bloodied gloves. Her hands contaminated the box and its contents with virus-laden blood. Jacques saw this and challenged her to first decontaminate her gloves. Any normal person would say "I'm sorry I made a mistake, thank you for putting me right", but she argued that she was "going to do it in a minute". Jacques quite rightly told her that she was to leave High Risk immediately. Laura is very passionate about the patients but it is incredible to see what a blind spot she has for safety and hygiene.

Russ and I reach the base hotel at quarter past seven in the evening, which is somewhat late for our in-between shift that started at ten o'clock in the morning. But my working day is not done yet. As soon as the Land Cruiser drives into the hotel compound, Eliseo walks up to meet me. Someone from the National Staff has had an accident with his motorbike and is waiting in the National Staff Clinic, across from the EMC. Eliseo asks me to turn around immediately and go back. I grumble. I'm tired after a long day, and could do with some dinner. Couldn't one of the expats that is still at the EMC see him? But no, apparently it could be serious, it can't wait etc, so I grab a cold drink from the fridge and jump back into the Land Cruiser.

Back at the Staff Clinic, I find one of the guards, John, lying down on the bench in the waiting room. I ask him to step into the clinic.

"So, what happened?" I ask, while starting my inspection of the injuries.

"I was riding my motorbike to work, to start my night shift. But suddenly there was a big snake on the road. I slipped and fell, and hurt my arm," he answers. John has some bruises and abrasions on his right arm, and a large bump on his forehead. Nothing's broken and he has not been unconscious. After I've checked that he doesn't have any possible Ebola-related symptoms, I gather some dressing material, and start cleaning his wounds.

John looks on with interest. Full of curiosity, he starts a list of questions like an interview. Where I'm from, what I do back home, whether I'm married, and if not whether I will marry him. My age is no object, he happens to be 40 years old too, so we would be perfect together. I thank him for his offer, but politely decline. We part good friends. His cheerful chat has cheered me up. He could easily have waited the half hour or so for my colleagues to finish their shift and tend to him, so there was really no need for me to go back to the clinic. I guess someone just made a wrong call. It is nearly nine in the evening before I get back to the hotel and dinner.

# Thursday, December 4

**Andy**
Today starts in a rather unusual way, I wake around half past seven, the sun peeks through the window to my left and illuminates the mosquito net that has protected me from my Nemesis once again. I wearily turn to my right, lift the net and step out. I walk the few steps to the bathroom for the much needed morning pee. I flush the loo and in a second I am jumping around the bathroom shouting, "f**k, sh*t, f**k"! As the toilet flushed, a frog wriggled out from under the rim and sat there as the water cascaded over it. I couldn't bear the thought of it dying in there so once my heart rate drops below 120, I root around till I find a bag containing some latex gloves (always good to carry some in my line of work). I then flush the toilet again and to my surprise I catch my quarry first time. I feel rather pleased with myself now that I have recovered from the original shock. I take it out to some bushes and let it go. First life of the day saved!

There is a different surprise when I arrive at the car to travel to the EMC at half past one. I was expecting to work with Laura at the EMC today. Well, it seems that yesterday she failed to follow the protocols for safe practice one time too many and is being sent home. So until her journey out of Sierra Leone can be arranged, she will have to stay at the base hotel.

More distressing for all of us is that another doctor is also being sent out. He is a kind and conscientious practitioner who made a foolish error yesterday. He put the needle from a cannula onto the floor instead of directly into the sharps disposal box. I can only assume he forgot to place the box before cannulating the patient. It was a mistake but my first thought is that sending him home was extremely harsh. As it turns out, he too was previously warned about staying in High Risk too long which makes this a second failure to comply with protocols MSF simply won't tolerate. I will miss this compassionate man and the project is losing a little bit of its conscience today. That said he can be proud of the amazing work he has done here and I know that he is a big enough person to look at what has happened and accept his mistakes.

For this reason, I leave the base feeling sad today.

# Friday, December 5

**Anna**

Andy and I have a day off together again, a good opportunity for another walk. This time, we walk in the direction of Kailahun, passing through the centre of the town. We take a path leaving town in the other direction, through thick green forest, and are cheerfully greeted by the locals along the way.

About an hour into our walk, while deeply engrossed in conversation, we pass by a remote homestead in the middle of the forest. Suddenly, a woman from the courtyard of the house starts yelling at us in Mende. We look up startled. There are several people sitting around the huts, who are watching us and smiling. The woman appears to be in charge. We can't understand her words, but it quickly becomes clear that she is jokingly and loudly berating us for our impoliteness of passing by without a greeting, or a word of admiration for her home. We are happy to make a cheerful show of greeting the family, and praising the beautiful homestead. We walk on amidst general laughter. On our way back, an hour or so later, we are prepared with our greetings and compliments as soon as the home comes in view.

Back in Kailahun town, we get into conversation with an older gentleman walking with a beautiful wood-carved traditional walking stick. He takes us along to introduce us to the Chief of Kailahun, who is sitting on the veranda of his house. We talk to him about the decreasing number of patients in the EMC, and how things are going in the right direction in his town. The old gentleman also walks with us to the town square, to meet the carpenter who made his walking stick. We tell him how much we admire his work, and end up ordering two hand-crafted walking sticks of our own. He promises that he will be able to make them by the end of next week, and that he will deliver them to the hotel.

Around one o'clock in the afternoon, we are back in the hotel. After lunch we decide to go out again, this time only a short stroll to the Ebola orphanage nearby. A group of children who have been discharged cured from the EMC and who don't have an adult relative to look after them are housed in two buildings run by the government. The children appear to be well cared for, and also have support from each other. The authorities try to find the best solution for the children, preferably returning them to relatives or at least to their home communities.

Andy and I recognise several of the children who have been discharged since we have been in Kailahun and they also recognise us. We play around a bit. I've brought a few gifts. In my home country, children are celebrating St Nicholas' day today, a children's holiday with gifts and traditional sweets. I've brought a bag of the traditional gingerbread cookies of the day. The children will have to wait to eat them later because we have arrived just before their meal. They can at least enjoy my other small gifts immediately. I come from a small village in the south of The Netherlands, called Liempde, that is famous for its poplars and its traditional wooden shoe factories, among other things. I had asked my parents, who still live in the village, to buy me a bag of small wooden shoe keyrings to take with me to Sierra Leone. When the clog maker heard that I would take them with me to Ebola-stricken Sierra Leone and why I wanted them he would not accept any payment but gave a large bag full of them. The children love their new treasures.

*Team effort*

A little bit of background on the people we are working and living with here. Something that most people do not realise is that there are more than just doctors and nurses working for MSF, despite only the doctors being featured in the name. There are so many more people from all over the world, all of who are indispensable. In the Kailahun project alone we have a Canadian psychologist who is in charge of a group of mental health counsellors from Sierra Leone who provide psychological support to our patients. An Australian epidemiologist, who collects all epidemiological data of the outbreak – where patients come from, where they were likely infected, how many patients survive, etc. One Dutch and one Haitian WatSan specialists, who are responsible for infection prevention and control, so everything to do with water and hygiene in the EMC, including the latrines, the water supply, the chlorination of water, cleaning of the clinic, and supervision of more than 100 national sprayers and hygienists. Every day, the EMC uses 260 litres of water per patient for cleaning, decontamination and hygiene. All of that water has to be transported to us by trucks. We have a technical logistician from Canada responsible for maintenance at the EMC. A Dutch logistician is responsible for supplies and transport, based at the hotel, and there is an administrative logistics expert from Kenya looking after the stores and purchases. We have a transport coordinator, responsible for all the Land Cruisers and the drivers. A British human resources manager is responsible for both expats and Sierra Leonean employees. There is a Canadian coordinator of finances.

Next, there is the important section of the Kailahun project known as the Outreach team. This includes three expats who are German, Dutch and Swedish. They coordinate the activities of large teams of health promoters and health counsellors, as we described before.

Then there are the managers: a manager of all medical activities in the EMC – an Italian nurse who is handing over this task to a Liberian replacement. He is responsible for the management of the national medical staff, making the rosters and taking care of practical medical issues in the hospital.

The role of Medical Team Leader has just been taken over by a British nurse who leads the medical work of the EMC as well as the Outreach team. The whole of the MSF project in Kailahun is under the charge of a project coordinator, the role taken by an experienced PC from Australia.

Two people who are not stationed in Kailahun but who have visited us in the past week are the Medical Coordinator of all MSF projects in Sierra Leone, who is from New Zealand, and the Dutch Head of Mission who is in overall charge of all the MSF projects in Sierra Leone.

In some projects, MSF will also employ their own lab-workers. In our Kailahun project, the Ebola tests are performed in a small laboratory run by Canadians, from the Canadian Public Health system. These three Canadians are also staying at our hotel.

This is a very large and complex operation, with so many different things going on at the same time. It is fascinating to watch this from close up.

# Saturday, December 6

**Anna**
Karimu, the CHO who normally runs the National Staff Clinic, is off today. So this shift, I spend about two hours in the Staff Clinic seeing local MSF employees with diverse physical complaints, including headache, skin rash, malaria. Luckily, no suspected Ebola. From tomorrow, one of our new expat doctors, Mark from South Korea, will take over the responsibility for 'National Staff health' from me. Now that Russ has ended his mission, I will take over as the contact person for 'expat health'. Any expat with health problems needs to get in touch with me. Because of the Ebola setting, where we want to trace any possible Ebola contamination as early as possible to enable a prompt repatriation, all expats have been instructed to report any health issues. Every case of diarrhoea, stomach ache, sleeplessness or itching.

I'm handed a box of medications to keep in my room, to hand out when needed. I also get training in yet another safety protocol: what to do if an expat reports to me with symptoms that might potentially be Ebola. The right procedure to isolate that person in his room, where to find the gear to improvise a small High Risk zone on the spot and how to approach him safely, in PPE, to review his health and draw blood, if deemed appropriate after consultation with the central MSF experts. Finally, what to do if the Ebola test turns out to be positive. I read through the protocol at least ten times to make sure I am prepared, just in case. I will keep my mobile phone religiously charged from now on, so that I can be contacted easily. Just before we arrived in Kailahun there had been an incident where one of the expats had a fever and the protocol had been put to use. Luckily it turned out to be malaria not Ebola. I sincerely hope I will not be called on to put this protocol into action.

From today, I will officially be the Clinical Focal Point in the EMC but we have decided to do away with the in-between shift. The number of expat doctors and nurses has significantly reduced (even faster than expected because of the recent dismissal of two doctors), and by now it is tricky to fill our working schedule, so I am going to continue on regular shifts.

Four out of the 12 tents in the EMC have been closed down and by the end of today only 18 patients are left, including three suspected Ebola (who likely have another cause of their symptoms), five patients in tent C4 we are still worried about, and ten patients who are convalescing. That is a very low number of patients for our EMC. To put it into perspective: the Kailahun EMC was one of the biggest Ebola management centres ever built, with the capacity to hold 96 patients. In past outbreaks, elsewhere in Africa, often only one EMC of about 20 beds was sufficient.

This morning, during the rounds in tent C4, 40-year old Amie is still a worry. Her breakfast is still in its carton, on the floor next to her bed, virtually untouched. When I squat down next to her bed to take her temperature I ask her how she is doing. She just kind of shrugs her shoulders and turns away from me.

When we persist in our questions, she just answers with a short yes or no, or even only a nod or shake of the head. We manage to get her to sit up and drink a bit, but it is difficult.

Something seems to be wrong. She does not have a temperature, and due to her IV fluids over the past few days she is not dehydrated anymore. Of course she is still weak, but her physical health seems to be really on the mend. She seems to have withdrawn within herself. The National Staff nurse who is with us suggests that perhaps she has a mental disorder. We hardly know anything about her, except that she was brought here by ambulance from Freetown in a very poor state. She could very well have some pre-existing condition that we are not aware of.

Back at the medical tents in the Low Risk zone, we discuss her case in the team. We get Sandra, our psychosocial worker from Canada, involved in the discussion as well. There is no immediate answer, but we decide to set up a meeting between Amie and the mental health counsellors that same afternoon. The team that goes into the High Risk zone around one that afternoon for an ORS and IV fluid round gets an extra task. From the Low Risk zone, I see Amie leaving the tent, supported by Andy and another nurse in PPE, very slowly walking towards the back of the clinic. In the visiting area, chairs are set up. Andy and the other nurse leave Amie on a chair, while Sandra and two local mental health counsellors in their regular street clothes sit down on chairs on the outside of the clinic, on the other side of the double fencing. A little over half an hour later, Amie returns to the tent. This time she walks more straight, and is only supported by one nurse. What's that, is she actually smiling?

Later, Sandra tells me the story of what happened to cause this miraculous change. Amie at first did not want to talk but only shrugged her shoulders and stared at the ground. After some skilful and persistent tactics, the counsellors finally managed to get through to her and to start a conversation. They found out that Amie did not really know where she was. She had been comatose on arrival. No one had thought to orientate her later and she had never asked. She had no contact with her family, she did not have a mobile phone. She had the feeling that her family had either abandoned her or had fallen ill themselves.

Luckily, she remembered her father's mobile phone number. When the counsellor called him on her mobile and put him on speaker, it became clear that Amie's family in Freetown had no idea where she had been taken. They thought that she had died. Her father burst into tears when he heard her voice and realised that she was still alive. Amie finally understood that her family had not disowned her. Only now did she reveal that she had four children of her own, whom she had never mentioned before, and who were all still healthy according to her father.

That conversation is what made the difference. Back at the tent, she now sat in a chair outside, she drank large cups full of ORS and asked for a banana.

That evening, the afternoon shift reports that Amie is now talking incessantly, she is laughing and she is playing the radio much too loudly. It looks like she is going to be all right.

*Psychosocial support*

MSF pays close attention to psychosocial support. Ebola and all the misery connected to it often leaves deep emotional scars. At our Kailahun project, Canadian expat Sandra, an experienced psychologist, works with a team of local employees, with experience in counselling. They try to support all the patients in the EMC. Explaining to the patients what is going to happen to them, finding out their problems, putting them in contact with relatives at home. Often, they are the ones who give the patients their Ebola test results. Getting the confirmation that yes, you have Ebola, and you will be transferred to the 'confirmed Ebola' tents is devastating news of course. But the good news that you don't have Ebola or that you are cured from Ebola, can sometimes have a deep impact as well. Apart from relief, there is often a feeling of guilt – why did you survive while others did not? Survivors may exhibit an increased sadness for all the others who died. Every patient who is discharged from the hospital has an exit interview with one of the counsellors.

A counsellor always attends our handover at two o'clock in the afternoon. If there is any patient that we are worried about, because of suspected mental problems or excessive stress, like Amie, we involve them immediately.

# Sunday, December 7

**Anna**
This morning when we turn up for the morning shift we are greeted by sad news. Osman has just passed away. This poor little boy had been so ill for such a long time, it is a wonder that he survived this long. Everyone felt for him, and it is the first thing everyone asked coming on duty: how is Osman doing? I write his name on the wooden stake that will mark his grave. A small symbolic gesture, the last thing I can do for him and his family.

Only one admission today: 49-year old Lovell fits the case definition for Ebola but I suspect it is more likely malaria. All in all, there are only 16 patients left in our EMC, and four of these are still very ill.

Amie is a different woman. She sits on a chair outside the tent and laughs and chats with the other patients. She is still weak but I have a good feeling that she will make it. One of her major complaints today was that her flip-flops were too small for her. That is easy to fix!

We are visited by a group from another aid organisation: expat doctors, nurses and a WatSan specialist, mainly from Australia, who are going to run a large EMC in Freetown. Under the guidance of an expert MSF expat nurse, who travelled with them, they will receive their first exposure to Ebola patients here, and to working according to the Ebola safety protocols. Who better to learn it from than MSF?

**Andy**

I check my emails first thing this morning and find a reply from Andrew Jones the MP for Harrogate:

*Hello Andy,*

*Thank you for the report from Sierra Leone.*
*Your journal entries are moving and clearly demonstrate the distressing circumstances under which you are working. It is difficult to imagine just how bad the situation is for the individuals concerned and indeed for those helping them.*
*I will certainly pass your email on to the Minister[4] and will get back to you as soon as I can.*
*Take care of yourself too.*

*Kind regards,*
*Andrew*

I am very sad to say that little Kadiatu is very poorly today. Her temperature is 40 degrees Celsius. I try in vain to put another cannula into her as we need to remove the current one that has been in for four days. We are concerned that the cannula itself could be acting as a focus for infection. Unfortunately I was unable to get another in so we are going to continue with the old one and try again tomorrow.

I took the blood of a 25-year-old man called Patrik this morning and commented on the fact that he looked very well. By noon we have the

---

4   Sometime later I did receive a reply from the UK Minister for International Development. However, it was a mix of statistics and evasion that in my opinion did not address the points I raised.

results, which confirm that he is cured. He is informed of this result as soon as possible. His already beaming smile widens as I tell him through Sarah's translation, "Patrik, your results are back and you have recovered enough to be discharged, you have beaten Ebola my friend."

At handover, I inform the afternoon staff that he can be discharged, the National Staff then swing into action and the plans are made for his departure. A new set of clothes and a towel are picked up and bagged by two staff in full PPE who then enter the High Risk area. They locate Patrik in the convalescence area and walk him to a shower block located next to the fence. Here he will have two showers, first with chlorine water, then with regular water. He will then change into his new clothes. Finally he will step through a gate in the fence and out of the EMC.

I have located myself opposite that gate with my camera. Here I will wait for him to exit the EMC, I plan to take a bunch of photos of this joyous occasion. I have already spoken to Patrik and have his permission to do this. I watch as he walks with the staff to the edge of the confirmed area. He then disappears into the shower and I spend a few minutes killing time by photographing the staff in their PPE. When he emerges I lift the camera and start snapping as he exits through the fence.

It takes me a moment to notice, and then I quietly whisper "f**king hell" to myself. I have just read the print on the donated T-shirt we have given to him. It strongly suggests that he participates in an act that is illegal in at least half a dozen African countries! The clothes we give out are donations from all over the world. No one has time or is even designated to check the print on them.

I walk with him to the 'hotel' from which he will head home in the next few days. As we walk, I recall being in Uganda in 2005. I had just returned from a week in the Displaced Persons camps and was tired but keen to get some exercise at the same time. I went for a run in the early evening and felt great for it. As I walked to cool down I passed a young man leaning on a wall looking like the cover of a 50 Cent album. He was being very cool and trying to look menacing. However this effect was somewhat undermined when he unfolded his arms to reveal a T-shirt that read 'Sometimes when I laugh I wet myself'. Yo Gangsta!

At the 'hotel' the Health Promotion staff present Patrik with his discharge certificate. I ask him to hold it up to cover his chest while I take some photos of him.

Later I return to the 'hotel' to give him an Italy football shirt to replace the offending garment. I think myself very funny when I suggest to Eliseo that in my opinion the Italy shirt was the more embarrassing.

# Monday, December 8

**Anna**

"Anna, is Anna there?"

I'm in the medical tent in Low Risk looking at some patient files, when Sandra's voice rings out from the direction of the road, around half past eight in the morning. I leave the tent and walk to the orange fencing that borders on the road. Sandra is standing there, with her mobile phone in her hand. She looks worried.

"Good morning, what is it?" I ask her.

"It's Janet, one of our mental health counsellors. You have met her, haven't you?" she responds.

I nod. I remember Janet, 46 years old, a friendly woman, very kind and patient in her contact with the patients.

"She has just called to tell me that she is not feeling well. I think it is bad, could you talk to her?" and she holds out the phone across the fence.

The mobile connection is not great, but good enough to make out that the signs are worrying. Janet has a fever, which started yesterday, with vomiting and diarrhoea. It rings all the alarm bells. I try to reassure her, while I'm already thinking of all the steps to take to get her over here to the clinic.

About an hour later, she arrives in an ambulance. I stay on the Low Risk side of the ambulance entrance to conduct the reception, while Mark, the South

Korean expat doctor, a local nurse and a sprayer go through the procedure. When the ambulance doors have been opened, Janet climbs out, supported by the nurse. How different it feels when it is someone you know, however slightly. She clearly looks ill, although she can still walk, with a little bit of support. I have a sinking feeling in my stomach, looking at her in triage. The full information we get from her in the triage hut only strengthens our suspicion that she may have Ebola, including fever and diarrhoea. Andy dresses in PPE to immediately collect a blood sample from her.

With only a little bit of extra work, the lab can run Janet's sample this same morning so we have the results early this afternoon. Unfortunately it confirms our suspicion: she, one of our own colleagues, has Ebola. It's a shock for everyone. As one of our employees, she gets a little hut by herself in the High Risk zone to the side of the clinic. We start her on all the supportive treatment available.

How did Janet become infected? Outside of the EMC, at home or somewhere else in her daily life? There is little Ebola in the province of Kailahun anymore. She lives just outside Kailahun town; we actually pass her house on our way to and from the EMC every day. That area has been free of Ebola for a few weeks now, as far as we know. So it is less likely although not impossible. Through her work then? The mental health counsellors at our EMC usually only speak to the patients from across the orange fencing, they very rarely go into the High Risk zone in PPE. She did make a visit to little Osman inside, in PPE, about ten days ago. Could it have happened then, was there some breach to the protective equipment, or a mistake in the undressing procedure? Or did she have contact with a patient in or outside the EMC in another way?

These questions keep everyone preoccupied, expats and National Staff alike. If it happened to her, could it not happen to any of us? There is no great concern that Janet herself has infected anyone at the EMC. She happened to have been on a holiday for the last five days, so hasn't seen any of her colleagues in that time and she only started showing symptoms yesterday. Also, MSF's strict 'no touch' policy is a clear advantage here. Even if she had worked up until this morning, the risk to her colleagues would have been negligible because no one touches anyone else nor shares personal items. Her family and her home will routinely be put in quarantine for 21 days.

Janet has a difficult decision to make before the afternoon is over. Just last week, a new small Ebola clinic has been opened in Freetown, that is especially meant for the care of medical and paramedical personnel from Sierra Leone who look after Ebola patients and who get the disease themselves. There is always this inequality that expat health workers who get infected with Ebola will be repatriated as soon as possible, where in a Western hospital setting the chances of survival are much greater than in an EMC like ours in Kailahun. Simply because there will be five nurses and one doctor for each Ebola patient, because more lab tests are available, because of the possibilities of kidney function replacement therapy in case of kidney failure, and artificial respiration if needed. The courageous Sierra Leoneans who work here, putting themselves at the same risk as the expats, have to be treated in the same EMC as their compatriots. Until now, that is. This new clinic is said to have almost the same level of care available as in a Western setting, including air-conditioning, lab tests and artificial respiration. So Janet gets offered a transfer to this new clinic in Freetown. It will mean saying goodbye to her family here in Kailahun, who won't be able to visit her or see her again while she is there because of the travel restrictions. If things go wrong, this would be their final farewell. Janet discusses it with her family and decides to grab the opportunity. She will be taken to Freetown by helicopter tomorrow, in a special isolation bubble.

That same afternoon, another memorable and complicated case arrives. Just after the two o'clock handover, the arrival of an unexpected ambulance is announced. I dress in PPE, together with a local nurse and a sprayer, to receive it. The ambulance has come from a small village in our province, and contains one patient without any papers or other information. When I open the back doors of the ambulance, I see a young man stretched out on his belly on the floor of the Land Cruiser, his bare feet towards us, wedged in between the bench and the stretcher. We call out to him, in English and in Mende, asking him to get up and move out of the ambulance. This is an Ebola-setting: our safety protocol demands that we try to avoid going into the back of the vehicle ourselves, unless it is absolutely unavoidable. The young man struggles to get up; it is painful to see how difficult it is for him.

After about five minutes of effort, he has got his upper body up from the floor, and is hanging face down over the bench at the side of the Land Cruiser.

Suddenly he starts to have severe convulsions all over his body, with very strong muscle spasms, his face down on the bench. He is at risk of choking on the foam that is coming out of his mouth. Instinctively, I move forward to help him. A loud shout from the direction of the Low Risk area calls me to attention: "Stop, don't go in! What is going on?"

I look in the direction of the shout. Jacques, our WatSan expat from Haiti, is standing at the orange fence, as the conductor of this ambulance arrival. From the sideline, he cannot see the inside of the ambulance. I explain to him what is happening, how the young man is in danger of choking to death because of his convulsions. This interruption is enough to bring me to my senses. This young man may well be severely ill with Ebola, meaning that he will be shedding a lot of virus. His uncontrolled muscle spasms and convulsions are a serious risk for our PPE inside the cramped ambulance, he could easily move my goggles or mask, or tear the overall, leading to exposure. So we have to remain outside until his convulsions have passed.

It is a dreadful interval of about ten minutes, standing there helpless, in our PPE, watching the young man suffering inside the vehicle. Jacques sends in two extra sprayers to help us, who were on their way into the High Risk zone for a cleaning round. By the time they join us, the patient seems to come out of his fit, only half conscious. Very carefully climbing into the ambulance, the two young male sprayers help manoeuvre the man out of the vehicle and onto a stretcher. The nurse and I then carry him to triage.

When we put the stretcher down on the floor, the young man briefly regains a little bit of consciousness.

I squat next to the stretcher. He manages to tell us that his name is Ishmael and that he is 14 years old. But that is all the information we ever get out of him. His whole face is swollen, especially around his lips and his eyes, resembling angioedema, a reaction often seen in allergies. I try to put him in the recovery position, because his airway is still threatened, but he is very agitated and hard to control. His body temperature is 37.9 degrees Celsius, so above the agreed threshold for fever for our Ebola case definition. I ask my colleagues in the Low Risk zone to prepare a dose of diazepam, to give him by injection, to try and control his agitation and muscle spasms. But I can feel that I should really be leaving. I have been in PPE for almost an hour, but it is more than just the time, I am exhausted and notice that I can't think properly anymore. Standing outside the ambulance waiting in the strong heat for the patient's convulsions to subside, carrying the full-grown teenager on the stretcher, and then the last ten minutes or so squatting down to examine him, and all in PPE, has taken its toll. Even just getting up from the squatting position I have to be careful not to fall over. I know that two other medics have almost finished dressing in PPE to come in to look after Ishmael. So I signal to the sprayer and nurse that we'll move out.

We walk along at a regular, controlled pace, careful as ever inside the High Risk zone. The sprayer, who has more energy left than I, asks us to stop at the decontaminating footbath between the suspected Ebola and probable Ebola areas. The footbath is almost empty, and he conscientiously wants to fill it with fresh chlorine water from a nearby tap. All I want to do is to move on to free myself from the overly hot and stuffy PPE, but I'm too exhausted to protest, and I figure it is quicker to let him do this chore than to explain why I want to walk on. However, while I am standing about waiting for a minute or so, one of the visiting expat nurses spots me from over the fence. She shouts out to me. She is all excited about the newly arrived patient and wants me to tell her all the details. All I can think is: not now! But I'm too tired to protest, so I satisfy her curiosity with about two sentences and then we move on, not paying any attention to her further questions.

When we finally reach the undressing tent I'm really nearing the end of my tether. I have never been so exhausted. I have trouble concentrating, and just stand in the tent like a zombie. The undresser realises the situation, and carefully coaxes me through the whole undressing procedure step by step. From outside the tent, Andy walks up while I'm still in the middle of the undressing. He starts to talk, but I sort of wave him away. I don't even have the energy left to explain to him that I can't talk now. He understands the situation and leaves, looking worried, so that I can concentrate on the task at hand. After the final washing of my hands, I stagger to a chair near the medical tent, and flop down with a bottle of water. This episode will remain with me as my single most exhausting time spent in PPE. Looking back, I stayed in PPE a bit longer than I should have.

To provide Ishmael with the best possible care in the circumstances, a sort of relay system has been set up. As I left High Risk, a fresh team of medics went in to carry him to a tent in the suspected Ebola area and to give him his first medication. By the time these people have to leave I am recovered from my dehydration and exhaustion and Andy and I go in together to assess the young man. Jacques completes our team. Now that our patient numbers have dropped, we can afford the time and effort to provide such care to our new arrivals.

Andy and I perform a reassessment of Ishmael's condition (what follows is a kind of technical medical description, for medically interested readers). His face and neck are grossly swollen, with heightened muscle tension and difficulty breathing, but he is still too alert to tolerate a mayo-tube (Guedel Airway) which is a tube inserted into the mouth to stop the tongue from falling back and blocking the air route to the lungs. Intermittently, he still experiences severe muscle spasms. His temperature peaks at 39.5 degrees Celsius. As we stand around his bed, he seems to be arching his back outwards (the medical term is opisthotonus). The muscle spasms and convulsions seem to get worse when we try to restrain the young man, to try to prevent him from hurting himself. On closer inspection he turns out to have an old wound on the sole of his right foot. Could it be tetanus? Neither of us has ever seen it in real life, but it would certainly fit with what we know of this deadly condition and he could have contracted it through the old wound on his foot.

Of course we cannot exclude Ebola until the tests come back negative. Alternatives that we review all seem less likely: Lassa fever, cerebral malaria, another kind of cerebral infection or cerebral tumour, a severe generalized allergic reaction, a kind of epilepsy, or a snake bite. Tetanus would not explain the angioedema of his face – could that be some kind of allergic reaction, perhaps to some form of traditional medication? Or just a traumatic effect of the journey in the ambulance, several hours, shaken about on the rough roads lying face down on the floor?

We don't have any tetanus immunoglobulin (a solution which contains a large volume of tetanus antibodies that can help fight the infection), which may sometimes help in cases of tetanus – though usually only in situations where patients can be kept alive by artificial respiration, and when given early enough. We decide to give medications for the treatable alternatives that we can think of, just in case it helps: steroids, adrenalin, antibiotics, anti-malarial drugs, muscle-relaxants (as much as we dare without impairing his breathing), glucose infusion and paracetamol to bring down his fever. Andy and I are kept busy with all the injections and infusions, while trying to keep the patient calm. We work well together, as we have found out in the past few weeks. Jacques very ably helps us out as much as he can, handing us equipment, decontaminating where necessary.

Unfortunately, there is no immediate positive effect. It is terrible to leave the teenage boy behind like that, on a stretcher in a big tent. We ask the other patient in the tent to keep an eye on the boy and ask him to let us know if something happens. It is already getting dark outside by this time. After we have emerged from the undressing tents, we share our thoughts on what we have just seen and done.

"Seeing you work like that, makes me want to become a nurse myself," says Jacques. Andy and I agree it is a good feeling to have made such an impression and to inspire our friend.

# Tuesday, December 9

**Anna**

We have changed the times of our morning shift. Because the number of in-patients and new admissions has dropped so much, there are far fewer blood samples to be drawn each morning. There is no need anymore to start the hour and a half before the National Staff day shift comes on, to profit from the lower temperatures and get that risky job done. So from now on, we'll start at eight in the morning, going through till about five in the afternoon.

No new admissions today. We are kept occupied by our existing patients. Janet has been prepared for her helicopter flight. Eliseo, who was leaving our Kailahun project anyway for Freetown, is travelling with her on the helicopter, as is Jacques, who plans to return after a brief rest and recuperation in the capital. We will miss them.

I'm doing the rounds in tent C4 today. This tent contains the most severely ill Ebola patients at this moment. A 20-year old man called Abu occupies the bed in the right-hand corner in the back of the tent. He has been very ill and restless for the past few days. The gangly young man already looked gaunt when he arrived last week. He was a patient in one of the last ambulances to arrive from Freetown, together with his brother and sister. This morning, when I squat down next to his bed, he does not really respond to my touch or my voice. He is still running a fever. There are no obvious signs of bleeding, and he does not seem to be troubled by hiccups as he was a few days ago. But he is very weak, and only semi-conscious. We have been treating him with IV fluids for the last few days, without a clear response. I fear the worst for him.

Out of the corner of my eye I see someone standing in the tent opening. I look up. It is Alpha, Abu's elder brother. Alpha is already at the convalescent stage, and is doing very well, as is their 14-year-old sister Mamani. Yesterday, Alpha told me that they have lost their parents and three of their siblings to Ebola before being struck down themselves. Alpha works as a builder in a suburb of Freetown, where Abu earns his living as a bike rider.

Now, Alpha looks at his brother on the bed, and then he looks at me, with a question in his eyes. I can guess what it is. I sadly shake my head, and tell him that I am very worried for Abu. More words are unnecessary. Alpha looks defeated.

Ishmael, the teenager who was brought in with convulsions yesterday, is clearly much worse this morning. He shows worsening neurological signs, and increased facial swelling. It is painful to see that every now and then he is conscious enough to realise his grave situation. Our outside contacts from the Outreach team have come up with little snippets of information about the background of the boy, although a lot remains a mystery. Apparently, he was playing with a group of children in a field when he suddenly fell down and started to have convulsions. At first he seemed to recover, but when the convulsions returned, the ambulance was called.

## Andy

I am on the afternoon shift today. I take the handover from the morning staff and Anna tells us that Ishmael has deteriorated significantly. My first job this afternoon is to go into High Risk Suspect Tent 1 to see him and assess his condition and comfort.

Once I am in PPE I enter High Risk with my National Staff colleagues and walk straight into the suspected Ebola area. I walk through the tied back flaps of the tent, look over to Ishmael's bed and I can see immediately that he is dead. I walk over to his bed, place a hand on his neck to check for a carotid pulse. I then check for breathing and pupil reactions. Nothing. Once this is done, I cover his body with a blanket and put a piece of paper with a cross on it on top as a marking for the hygienists who will come in next and move him to the mortuary. Ishmael age 14 died alone in a tent in Kailahun, December 9, 2014. He mattered.

This evening we have a visitor. An MSF executive has come to visit Kailahun EMC. This man is very experienced with MSF and has worked on numerous missions in many different contexts. In my book, this in itself commands a degree of respect. Respect however is not unconditional and is easily lost. The whole team chuckles as one when this executive seriously begins to complain about a lack of hot water for his personal use at our base hotel. He isn't satisfied until he has got his hands on our one kettle to heat water for his bathroom. Not one of the team has even mentioned this, it is a total non issue to all of us and then someone who has probably more field experience than the lot of us put together makes it into a big deal. We spend the rest of the evening trying to out do each other with ludicrous suggestions of luxury that we 'need' to make the project tolerable. I want PPE with circulating liquid nitrogen coolant and a hovercraft to get me to the EMC as that road is just so bumpy!

# Wednesday, December 10

**Andy**

I am very sad to say that little two-year-old Kadiatu is not drinking or eating anything like enough to sustain her. After a long discussion the team has taken the big decision to place a naso-gastric (NG) tube and feed her via this. An NG tube is inserted through the nose, to the back of the throat, down the oesophagus (the food pipe or gullet) and into the stomach. Liquid food can then be passed down the tube to hydrate the patient and provide nutritional support.

The insertion of these tubes can be tricky; there is always the risk that the tube may be passed into the lungs by accident. The act of inserting an NG tube in a patient with Ebola is in itself very risky. The tube is passed through what is a very vascular area, which means it has a rich blood supply. If any damage is sustained and the patient starts to bleed they may not stop. Ebola as one of the viral haemorrhagic diseases interferes with blood clotting so that any kind of bleed can be life threatening.

To insert the tube, we move Kadiatu from the tent to a space near to the fence between High and Low Risk. It is well lit but also has some shade. I sit opposite Janet, one of the National Staff medics. She lifts Kadiatu and places her upright on her knee. I have all of the equipment I will need in a bag on my lap. I take out the NG tube and measure a couple of landmarks.

One is the distance to the back of the throat and the other the distance to the stomach. I then lubricate the tube, and prepare to insert it.

"I'm going to start now, Janet," I say quietly. I stroke Kadiatu's listless face once and then lift the tube to her right nostril. I have to focus on the job and try to detach my mind from how sorry I feel for this small child. I slide the tube to the first marker. She doesn't respond to this. While I should be pleased that the insertion hasn't upset her I am concerned that she is so unresponsive to what is often quite an upsetting procedure for a child. I continue to insert the tube to the second marker, which indicates that the tube should be in her stomach. I draw back on the syringe, which I have attached to the NG tube. Immediately, about 30ml of bile appears in the syringe which goes some way to confirming that the tube is in her stomach. Normally I would run this over some litmus paper and confirm a strongly acid fluid. Sadly we don't have any litmus paper and so I double check with what's called the bubble test. It is not considered very reliable these days but it's the only test option available. I blow about 40ml of air down the tube while listening for a bubbling noise over the stomach with a stethoscope. I hear the bubbles despite having to put the stethoscope earpieces into my ears on top of my PPE hood. Once I am convinced of the tube's position, I tape it into place and then give the little girl 120ml of F-100, a special therapeutic milk.

Before I leave the high-risk area, I ask Amie if she would be prepared to watch Kadiatu and to let the staff know if there are any problems. She is happy to do this, however little Miss Kadiatu still managed to pull the tube out half an hour later. I will re-insert it tomorrow and this time I am sad to say she will be having some little boxing gloves made with cotton wool and bandages to try to stop her pulling it out. This feels mean but it could save her life.

**Anna**
Near the end of the afternoon shift, at almost half past seven, there is news of the arrival of another ambulance. I'm going to dress in PPE to receive it. I ask for a volunteer from the WatSan team to accompany me. The young people are understandably not very eager; whoever goes in is likely to miss the bus transport home that inexorably leaves at a quarter past eight and waits for no one. For most of them, this means a long walk home after the day's work. But one of the sprayers, Sam, is willing to help out.

It is an ambulance from a village a few hours away in Kailahun province. This time, we uniquely have a little bit of information on the patient beforehand. Earlier this afternoon we received a phone call from a colleague on the Outreach team. This particular village had been in quarantine for some time because of earlier cases of Ebola. The community is not very welcoming to outsiders and has been known to conceal people with symptoms for fear of them being taken away and the quarantine being continued. They still put their full trust in traditional healers. A few weeks ago, the old chief of the village had died from Ebola, as well as his wife, followed by their daughter-in-law. About two weeks ago, the chief's adult son had been brought to our clinic, severely ill with Ebola, and had died within 24 hours. The villagers have not reported any new cases of illness in their midst since that time. But this morning, when a couple of health promoters visited the area on purpose to check things out, they spotted a young boy of about four years old who appeared to be showing signs of illness. It was the chief's grandson.

After Sam has sprayed the back doors of the ambulance and I have opened the doors, we indeed see a small boy sitting on the bench on his own, although he looks to be more like nine years old. I ask him his name. He shyly replies, "Brima." The boy is a bit shaky on his feet, but can walk to the triage hut by himself. Before we can start to question him, I have to help him to walk to the nearby latrine, because of his severe diarrhoea. Back on a seat in the triage hut, we give him a bottle of water and a packet of biscuits. We try to put him at his ease as he is so young and so ill. It must be a very frightening experience to be suddenly transported, all alone, to this world of people in PPE, that he has probably only heard bad rumours about in his community, and where his father went to a couple of weeks ago, never to return. Brima does not have a fever. Around his waist is a knotted rope, a sign that a traditional healer has seen him. His own story, upon questioning, is that the only one in his family who has been ill is a brother who had a bout of vomiting and diarrhoea a week or two ago but has since recovered spontaneously. He doesn't say a word about his parents and grandparents dying of Ebola. So it is good that we have some inside information because this has to be the same boy.

In the evening, the outside temperature has cooled down to an agreeable level, so I keep going for longer in PPE (except for somewhat fogged goggles that deteriorate my vision). Sam and I continue to take Brima inside the High Risk zone to a bed in one of the 'suspected Ebola' tents. I get him some clean trousers because he has not been able to stop his diarrhoea during the lonely hours-long ambulance trip. Sam explains the do's and don'ts for patients inside the EMC to him in Mende. I hand the boy his first medication and a cup of ORS to drink. We cannot safely give patients in the High Risk zone IV fluids in the night but he will certainly be a good candidate for that in the morning. That brings us to the end of our hour.

By the time we get undressed and ready to go, it is past half past eight. As expected, sprayer Sam and his colleague who volunteered to decontaminate the ambulance have missed the bus. Andy and I offer them a seat in the MSF Land Cruiser that is ready to take us back to the hotel, and drop the young men off somewhere along the way in Kailahun town.

# Thursday, December 11

**Andy**

Happy birthday dear Tracey. It has been a tough time apart. One month is not long in the scheme of things but I have missed her very much. This has been compounded by very poor communication options. On my first mission back in 2005 contact home was via text-only emails for six months. These days however we are somewhat spoilt by access to Skype in most missions. It's true that you expect what you are used to and I fully expected to be able to talk to Tracey on Skype pretty much every night. This hasn't worked at all; the internet connection has been at best sporadic.

Today I am working from eight till five with Elisa, a newly arrived Dutch nurse who seems very pleasant. It appears that I am now considered a grizzled veteran.

We arrive at the EMC and Elisa and I attend handover and then change into PPE to take the morning bloods. By now there are few patients in the EMC and we only have five samples to take. This allows me time to show and reinforce my methodical approach to blood taking. I smile at one point as I say to her, "No one survives an Ebola needle stick injury, Elisa." I am quoting Eliseo's words to me from a month ago. I wonder who he was quoting?

After this I talk to the other medics about the plan for Kadiatu. It is agreed that as we cannot get venous access and she cannot drink, that re-insertion of the naso-gastric tube is appropriate. I think we all feel some degree of reservation about this knowing the inherent dangers. As with many things in medicine it is a risk versus benefit issue. In this case the decision almost makes itself, Kadiatu will die unless we start to rehydrate her very soon.

I make up the F-100 milk and rehydration salts and then Elisa and I again enter High Risk to reinsert the tube. Poor Kadiatu is pretty much the same as yesterday, listless, dehydrated and very, very sick. I know that this is the last chance to save her and although I don't like the idea of putting cotton wool and bandages on her hands, we have to retain this tube. The tube re-insertion is straightforward and again I give the first fluids after checking the position. I feel awful as we leave her with Amie as she is irritated by the presence of the tube and her tiny hands covered in bandages move up to her face before flopping down again as fatigue and illness overwhelm her.

Brima, the young boy Anna admitted yesterday has, as suspected, tested positive for Ebola. He is in worse shape than last night so we insert an IV cannula in advance of his needing one urgently if he stops drinking. The theory there is that he will be harder to cannulate if his condition worsens and he becomes significantly dehydrated. Sheku, one of the nurses, helps me sit him up and we give him a drink and some medication that is due. He struggles to swallow the meds but manages slowly. It is always difficult inside High Risk as we have a lot to do each time we enter but each patient needs a lot of time as every action or intervention is slow and difficult for them. The key is simply accepting that you can only do so much and that there will be another team going in soon after who can pick up on incomplete jobs.

We leave the tent after helping Brima and I enter the undressing tent to begin the process of removing my PPE. Outer gloves first and then my apron. This is secured by a waist level elastic band with a hook that passes through an eye. As I unhook this metal fastening, which is somewhat rusty from its frequent chlorine baths, it catches my PPE and opens a two-centimetre tear in my overall near to my right hip, exposing a little bit of the scrubs underneath. As I have been sprayed all over with chlorine solution at the start of the undressing procedure, and that area of my overall is highly unlikely to have any contamination from the patients we have just seen, it is probably not a big deal. I continue with my undressing routine as per normal. I will change my scrubs anyway but will report this incident to the Medical Team Leader. We need to look at these fastenings as it has been mentioned as a possible risk before now.

When I am finished in High Risk, I walk round to the convalescence area where I take some photos of the little boy from Freetown called Musa, who has lost most of his family to Ebola. He was understandably very low of mood at one point as well as very sick physically. He has recovered remarkably. The psychosocial care team has worked with him intensively and he has thrived. He shows me his drawings in a book that was given to him by Eliseo. He has drawn pictures of the things that he has seen while he has been an inpatient. MSF Land Cruisers, United Nations helicopters that have flown over, some armed men who accompanied the President of Sierra Leone when he visited the EMC a couple of weeks ago. His pictures are very good and I take photographs of them for him. When he is discharged, he can take nothing with him – everything he owns will be burned, including his book. I take the pictures so that we can print them out for him and give them to him when he leaves the EMC. His beaming smile lights up the convalescence area. We did his blood test today and although he is clinically cured his blood viral levels are still not quite there. We will check his blood in three days and I am confident he will be ready for discharge then.

The last thing I do before I say goodbye is to throw Musa a bag containing a new set of clothes. In return I receive my fix of that wonderful smile!

# Friday, December 12

**Anna**
Friday morning shift, starting with the handover as usual. CHO Tommy has been on duty the past night. Little Kadiatu, the two-year old girl, has been very restless all night. She kept crying. Tommy says that he eventually had to remove the naso-gastric tube because it seemed to be troubling her a lot. Andy responds angrily. That naso-gastric tube was put in very carefully again, yesterday, and they had wrapped the little girl's hands in bandages just to make sure she would not be able to pull it out this time. "Of course she doesn't like the tube, no one does, but it's her only chance for survival. She's not able to eat or drink enough herself. Without that tube she's going to die!"

Tommy is taken aback by Andy's outburst, but persists in his opinion that they didn't have a choice. Andy is not really listening anymore. He has already started to gather the things needed to give the little girl a naso-gastric tube for a third time.

Kadiatu arrived in our clinic on November 30, in an ambulance from far away. Andy and I are about the last remaining expats who were around when she arrived and who remember what state she was in. The little girl was so weak, her mouth was bone-dry, with encrusted blood on her lips. It was painful to watch, let alone what she must have felt herself.

She was not even able to cry or really respond to her surroundings. After a few days of IV fluids and medication for her pain and nausea, she seemed to improve a little. With special care she could drink a little or eat a few spoonfuls of prepared food. She regained the ability to moan and cry. But she remained very weak. She had recovered from the worst of the dehydration but she was still struggling to battle the Ebola virus.

Directly after the handover, Andy takes the equipment into the High Risk zone. He is accompanied by Elisa, a local nurse and a sprayer from the WatSan team. To profit from better light and air, they carry the little girl out of the tent, bed and all, and put the stretcher in the open space next to the double fencing separating High and Low Risk zone near the medical tent. But it quickly becomes clear that the girl is not doing well. She is dyspnoeic, struggling for each breath of air, and is restless because of pain. Andy and Elisa sit down in chairs on both sides of the bed, and call to me. I walk over to the fencing.

Andy looks at me from behind his goggles. "It's not good," he says, but I can see that myself, even from the safe 2m distance. Few words are needed. It is too late for Kadiatu, she is dying. I cross the Low Risk zone to the medical tent and quickly prepare a syringe with medication to give the little girl some relief from pain and the feeling of choking. I hand it to Andy across the fences.

Here we are. Elisa and Andy dressed up in PPE, aside the bed of the dying girl, both holding a little hand in their big double gloved hands. I am in the green scrubs, on a wooden stool in the Low Risk zone at the other side of the fence. Elisa, who knows that we have been trying our best to save this girl for the last two weeks, offers to change places with me so that I can go inside. But I do not want to intrude.

The work in the EMC continues around us. Steve, our logistics expert, is doing some repairs to the tents nearby in High Risk. I move away to the medical tent to prepare medication for other patients, for my colleagues who are doing the rounds. The WatSan team is busy on a cleaning round inside High Risk. Everyone knows what is going on. Death has been part of the daily life of our EMC for months.

A little while later, Andy and Elisa call me over again. Time to make a plan. The hour in PPE is almost up for them, and we don't want to leave Kadiatu on her own at this time. There is not much we can do for her anymore but at least we can make sure she is not alone at the time of her death. No one knows how long that will be, however if we set up a relay system she does not need to be left alone. I get to action. First thing is to find some buddies to take inside with me. I explain to them what the object will be: to sit with the dying girl – because I want volunteers who are prepared for that. Liliane, a young nursing aid that I liked working with on previous occasions, offers her help. Joined by a young female sprayer we dress up in PPE and walk through the EMC to Kadiatu's bed. Andy's buddies of the morning have just left for the undressing tent. Andy remains at the bedside and I sit down on the other side of the bed. After a brief discussion we decide to give the girl some extra medication because she is still somewhat restless.

How small she is, how lovely and beautiful her little face. Someone back at her home – perhaps her mother – has lovingly put lots of small braids in her hair, each of them has a colourful rubber band. I take her small hand in my big hand, protected by two layers of gloves.

In the Low Risk zone, Albert walks over, the expat nurse who has just become the Medical Manager of the EMC. He warns Andy that his time in PPE is up: he has been inside for more than an hour, and rules are rules. Andy looks at me. I can see that he wants to object. It is not likely to be long for Kadiatu and he does not want to leave her but there are numerous people around and he can't undermine Albert's authority. We all know how important it is to work safely inside an EMC, and that means we have to comply with the safety protocols, no matter how difficult it is in these circumstances. Andy casts a final glance at Kadiatu and then rises and moves away to the undressing tent. As soon as he is back in the Low Risk zone he sits down on the stool across the fence, a couple of metres away.

I remain behind with the little girl, with Liliane. I hold Kadiatu's small hand in my one hand, and with the other I alternately stroke her hair, or her face. I softly murmur some words to her I don't even remember what. It doesn't matter.

It isn't that long after Andy's departure, I think it must have been about 20 minutes, when Kadiatu peacefully drifts off and her breathing stops. I stroke her little face for a last time. Andy rises from his chair and walks away without a word, clearly emotionally charged. My eyes are filled with tears, behind the double layers of glasses and goggles.

Liliane and I put a note with Kadiatu's patient number and a cross on the bed, and cover the little girl's body with a blanket. On my way to the undressing tent I change my mind: there is something urgent to do first. I walk to the tents for convalescent patients to find Amie, who has been looking after Kadiatu for the last few days at our request. The few patients that remain in the EMC have kept their distance for the past hour. I want to tell Amie that the little girl has passed away. She has a right to hear it from us and not find out accidentally.

Amie can clearly feel it coming, when she sees Liliane and me walking up to her. In the middle of the big empty tent, I tell her what happened. I put my gloved hand on her shoulder. Her reaction is very emotional. I do not really need Liliane's translation, it is clear enough without that. She is sad and angry. Kadiatu had been doing badly all night and Amie had been very worried. She so did her best to look after her. I try to reassure her: she has done everything that she could, she did a good job looking after the girl but the Ebola was too strong for her. Amie turns around and walks away from us.

This is one of the few times that I am hardly sweating when I undress. Despite everything that happened, it is still early morning and therefore still cool and this time our efforts were more emotionally than physically taxing. I emerge from the PPE with tears in my eyes. In the medical tent I find out what Andy has been doing. He has prepared Kadiatu's burial stake. He has neatly written down her name, age, patient number, home village and date of death and at the corner, he has lovingly drawn a colourful little flower with red petals.

Everyone is affected by Kadiatu's death, despite the fact that we deal with death on a daily basis here. That she was so young and all on her own in the EMC is a factor but she was not unique in that; that was true for so many other patients in the past few weeks. It is because we have been able to surround her with so much care. This time, we were able to make sure that she was not alone at the moment of her death, that someone was there who cared for her. It reminds us of all the other patients in the past weeks for whom we have not been able to do that; who we were only able to give some extra painkillers but then had to leave because we had to move on to the next patient, who were then found dead a few hours later.

For Andy and me, Kadiatu's death becomes a symbol for all the other patients who didn't make it. Her memory is important and her life is not inconsequential. Her story must be told, without it she is just a name on a wooden stick fading in the Sierra Leone sun and she was so much more.

Back in the medical tent, we go through the registers together to find out how many patients have been here since our first working day in the EMC on November 18. On that day there were 77 patients in the EMC and, over the weeks since then, 87 patients have been newly admitted. Out of those, 47 have died in Kailahun in the four weeks. There have been 75 Ebola patients who have been discharged cured. (We didn't count how many patients were discharged as 'non-case' since they were Ebola negative.)

After lunch, Elisa, Andy and I take a walk from the EMC to the Moa river crossing that marks the border with Guinea. It is good to take our minds off the sadness of the morning for a little while. The border has been closed for months because of Ebola and the offices are abandoned. It is a beautiful spot, quiet and serene. Along the way, we pass a small hamlet of about five huts. The people are all outside, working and chatting. A few girls suddenly call out my name! I am amazed: how do they know who I am? It turns out their big sister is employed in the EMC. I've chatted with her a few times, and she has pointed me out to her little sisters.

That evening is Andy's last in Kailahun, his mission ends tomorrow. Intense and weird days here, with such vivid experiences.[5]

---

5  Andy: Anna describes the events of today perfectly. I would add little to the story of dear Kadiatu's last day except to lay my emotions open. I was devastated when this little girl died. She came to personify the Ebola outbreak for us. I will never forget the time I spent sitting with her in the EMC on that last morning. I felt empty inside as I watched her young life slip away. Moving forward in the timeline of this book, since my return home I dedicate my presentations about Doctors Without Borders to her memory. As of July 2015 I find myself emotionally fragile whenever I talk about her.

# Saturday, December 13

**Anna**

I'm on morning shift today, so leaving the hotel early. That's good as Andy is leaving, and I don't like saying goodbye. We've been through so much together in the past few weeks. I was in awe of him at the start, as one of those very experienced MSF-ers with a very adventurous background. He has taught me a lot and we quickly found out at that we work very well together, needing few words to get a job done, despite our different personalities and backgrounds. I will miss him and the project will not be the same for me without him.

Little Brima, the new boy in C4, is in a bad way this morning with a lot of pain. He has deteriorated, despite IV fluids and medical treatment. When we go to change his diaper, it is full of bloody diarrhoea, he squirms from pain. His abdomen is very stiff and painful to the slightest touch. He must have had internal bleeding. We work to get him as comfortable as possible, very carefully giving him a wash, administering morphine and other medication. I sit down next to him for 10 minutes or so, while I stroke his head and face, and murmur softly to him, while he lies with his eyes closed. This quietens him, until the medication starts to work. It is not advanced medical care but it is all we can do.

In the evening, when the afternoon shift returns to the hotel, I learn that Brima has died. He remained practically unconscious until his death. I'm glad of the fact that he was no longer conscious, and am also glad I was there in the morning to give him medication and to stroke his head until it started working. He was a cute boy, although likely a naughty wild one in everydaylife. I guess by the end of my time here, at the end of this week, we will know the (Ebola-related) fate of all of these patients.

**Andy**
My final morning in Kailahun. My final day in Sierra Leone and it's going to be a long one. I am up at half past six, as I want to see the people who are heading to the EMC. I catch up with the Land Cruisers just before they leave the Base. It is tough to say goodbye but I already treasure the time I have spent with them here. Saying goodbye to Anna is especially difficult. She has been amazing. She came to this mission as a first timer with MSF and she has put some of the experienced MSF people to shame with her level headed and balanced approach. I enjoyed walking with her and chatting about the patients. She feels intensely about them. That is not to say for a moment that the others didn't, I just spent more time in both the EMC and socially with Anna than anyone else.

The helicopter that will take me to Freetown lands at a nearby football pitch about half past eleven. I therefore have plenty of time to say goodbye to the base staff. I have a chat with a guy called Albert who runs the radio room. Albert is a budding artist and has drawn some pictures with various messages about Ebola. Keeping busy is good as it allows me little time for panic. This will be the first time since the Gulf War in 1991 that I have been in a helicopter. In fact, I vowed I would never fly in one again. However, my alternatives were limited for the journey to the capital. Eight hours in a vehicle with the chance of delays on the abysmal roads or 10mg of Diazepam and a drug-induced haze to get me onto the helicopter for a two-hour flight that only gravity could ruin.

There are eight people on the flight out of here today. Some are from the headquarters of MSF in Sierra Leone but there are others from organisations such as the World Food Programme and the Red Cross. One passenger, a very efficient and knowledgeable woman seems to feel that she has to manage everybody all of the damn time. She can't stop herself from organising us so I just walk away from the group as we wait for the aircraft to arrive. I don't really know any of the people flying out and quite frankly I don't feel very sociable. My mind is on the people in the project I am about to leave behind.

The helicopter arrives in a cloud of dust. I hide behind a 'Cruiser' but still manage to look like I have acquired an instant tan. The rotors on the large Russian flagged UN helicopter come to a stop, the dust settles and we walk from the touchline of the football pitch to the door. I board and find a seat next to the window on the starboard side of the aircraft. Five minutes later and Kailahun is behind me along with the happiness and the heartbreak of the last month. I know I will never be back here but I also know that this place will never leave me. I watch as the town gives way to a green carpet of trees and then remarkably I fall asleep.

We arrive in Freetown about half past one and are taken to the main MSF office. There is a bath available here albeit with cold water. I enjoy a refreshing shower and lose my dust tan immediately. Afterwards I find a space away from the busy HQ staff and sit down to read my emails and my eyes are drawn immediately to one from Anna who tells me that Brima has died.

In the evening, four people including myself who are leaving on tonight's flight join a number of headquarters staff at a restaurant on the beachfront called Roy's. It is a lovely place anyway but after the relatively basic and somewhat repetitive food we had in Kailahun, hummus and a pizza are heavenly.

After the meal I walk out of the restaurant and straight onto the beach. I take ten minutes to walk along the sand. I feel a little sad. I guess there are many reasons. I'm leaving a place where my job, though emotionally and physically difficult was at least clear, straightforward and fulfilling. I am leaving a team of both National Staff and expats who have impressed me in so many ways with their compassion and dedication, add to that new found friendships. Perhaps most of all I am leaving a place where so many tears have been shed both privately and in the last day or two openly and without shame. When something means so much it is always going to be painful to leave. The crashing of the waves draws me back to the present and I return to the restaurant.

We leave Roy's about nine o'clock and are taken by car to the water taxi terminal. Processing here is fairly slick and we are not waiting around for long before we board the boat to make the 30 minute trip to Lungi and on to the airport.

It seems like only a few days since my arrival at the airport. This time there is no mystery in the chlorine hand wash points and the frequent temperature checking. I fill in a two-page questionnaire about my recent work and travel before joining a massive queue for check in. There is little option but to 'people watch' here and there is no shortage of subject matter, hundreds are waiting for flights. Concerns about people travelling from Ebola affected areas seems to have been dealt with rationally. There is little to worry about as long as a person is well and not exhibiting symptoms and this appears to be well monitored.

It takes two and a half hours to get through check in, however the delay is not a problem, I fly about three o'clock in the morning which gives me about two hours to wait in departures.

# Sunday, December 14

**Anna**

Only ten patients are left in the EMC this morning. Amie's blood test came back negative today – she is very happy to be discharged, finally able to leave the EMC and all its bad memories behind!

I thought of a new trick to keep ten-year-old Musa occupied – he is getting bored now that his health is improved and he is just waiting for his blood test to be OK. From the Low Risk zone, across the fence, I set him assignments to draw. A car, a goat, a banana tree. Each time he quickly runs away to his tent or to the convalescent area to work on the challenge and when he is finished he returns to the fence and calls out for me to admire the result. The car is good, the goat is OK. The banana tree is so good that I suspect he may have secretly had some help from his friend Alpha, who has a good hand at drawing.

Abu is still going (I will not say 'strong'); his brother Alpha was declared cured today but is staying on to wait for him. The two other women in convalescence are well, but have to wait for their Ebola virus levels to go down. Michael is still showing strange behaviour. Today we found out that the strange package in tape that he carries with him is his mobile phone closely wrapped around with medical tape; he seems to want to protect himself from receiving messages. The swelling of his feet is getting less, and his viral load is only just measurable now, so he will be OK for discharge in a few days.

**Andy**
Half past five in the morning and I am now back in the uninspiring surrounds of Casablanca airport. It is cool and raining outside which adds to my dislike of this place. This time however I am prepared for the fact that they have zero food for vegans and I have some provisions with me. I don't leave for Amsterdam for another five hours but I feel quite smug as I open up my bag and take out a fully charged laptop and some nice food, sit back and start to watch *Clash of the Titans*.

It is an unremarkable flight to Holland, I watch a couple more films and doze a little but find it impossible to sleep properly.

I arrive at Schiphol Airport (Amsterdam) mid afternoon. It is odd that all four of my missions have ended in December and all before Christmas. It is wonderful to see the Christmas decorations looking so beautiful. I find myself thinking about Kadiatu and how this little girl of two years should have seen Christmas lights, she should have received a present and she should have grown up. In my mind I see her face as I walk past the lovely lights.

I remain contemplative as I sit in the shuttle bus heading towards the city, looking out of the rain-spattered window at the streetlights. I think about the solar streetlights in Kailahun, I had never seen that in an African town before. I felt a longing to be back there and a sense of loss at my departure. I miss the ubiquitous red soil of Africa already.

The shuttle drops me at the Lancaster Hotel and I trudge to reception feeling jaded. I check in and make it to the room where I unpack a few things before lying on the bed and have a couple of hours sleep.

At eight o'clock I cross the road to the rather posh De Plantage Restaurant where I order a lovely vegan meal and a bottle of champagne. I was mulling over the decision to do this before I arrived in the city. I wanted to do something nice, as this has been a good mission. I feel have been effective and have made a positive contribution. I think these things can be celebrated and don't believe that wearing sackcloth and ashes about the injustices of the world changes anything.

I enjoy the meal but equally I enjoy just sitting in this lovely place looking out into the Amsterdam night. The garden at the back of the restaurant has some quite beautiful white Christmas lights. This time I am able to appreciate the scene without memories of Kailahun upsetting me. I relax with the remainder of the champagne before leaving for the hotel about midnight.

I look forward to tomorrow evening when I should be back with Tracey and my Mum and Dad, this has been a hard time for all of them and it will be an emotional homecoming.

# Monday, December 15

**Andy**
So, the lesson for today: if you want a leisurely breakfast don't forget to set auto update on the time zone settings on your phone/alarm. I wake at eight o'clock and am casually preparing for the day until I glance at my watch and realise it is in fact nine o'clock – the time I am due at the office. I shower, dress and eat breakfast at speed before leaving the hotel at nine thirty.

I arrive at the MSF office about ten minutes later, sweating profusely and looking anything but calm and rested and ready for a day's debriefing. There are a number of people to see today and I begin with staff health. They want to talk about my physical state and if there are any issues. I explain about the two minor PPE 'breaches'; one where my goggles slipped and exposed a small area of skin on my face which was noticed immediately and I left High Risk, the other when a hook on my apron strings tore a 2cm hole in my yellow overall. I make it very clear that these were incredibly low risk events and I had reported them immediately. The staff explain the Public Health England policy on returnees from Ebola areas. I am to be off work until 21 days (the incubation period of Ebola) has elapsed. Within that time I will be self monitoring my temperature and general health and ringing the public heath people with updates daily. I will receive further guidance and appropriate equipment when I arrive home. It all sounds very thorough.

Later in the morning I go to talk to the psychosocial team. I immediately recognise the lady who is going to conduct my debrief, having met her after my last mission in South Sudan. She is very kind and I recall her being easy to talk to. Five minutes later I am in floods of tears having described the deaths of Kadiatu and Osman, the little boy who died along with his father in the EMC. It is a painful discussion but one that I need to have at this early stage. I know that there will be a lot of interest in the events of this last month when I return home and I have to be able to talk openly about it. I talk to her for the best part of an hour and leave with a contact card should I need to be in touch after my arrival in Yorkshire.

I finally leave the MSF office about two o'clock. I head to the pub across the street from the hotel where I sit and enjoy a beer and think back to mid November when I sat in this place with Alessandro. So much has happened in that short time. It seems almost like a dream. My surroundings in this bar feel like a world away from Kailahun. In the words of a photographer I met in Uganda in 2005, "Same world mate, just different breaks."

I take the shuttle bus to Schiphol airport about six o'clock, implementing my usual pre flight plan of sedation en route (it works particularly well on top of a Belgian beer) and wait for the flight to Leeds.

After an uneventful flight the city lights of Leeds come into view and provoke a mixed bag of feelings.

I am nervous about returning home. In many ways I have been living a very straightforward life for the last month. I would go to work in what was of course a difficult area but when I left I would just return to base, have a chat, maybe go for a walk and that was it. Back home there is the complexity of my "normal" life to cope with. I have hardly spoken to Tracey over the last month due to technical constraints, my contact with everyone has been via email as and when I could. People have been very understanding but I know that there will be expectation that I will be around and willing to open up about the mission when I return home.

Conversely, there are people who do not want to see me when I return due to fear about my being a 'carrier' of Ebola. Before I left I posted a number of entries on my website and other social media with factual information about the virus and the risk to people from returnees. Despite this, one friend decided that he wanted to postpone a meeting we had planned for late December. I will of course accept people's right to decide such things but I will continue to try to spread the word: if I am well and have no symptoms I cannot pass Ebola to you or your family.

I make my way from the aircraft to passport control, as I walk the corridors I see a number of signs asking people 'Have you been to West Africa?' and listing symptoms of Ebola. It was made very clear to me in Amsterdam that we are to be totally open about where we have been and what we have been doing. As I near the front of the queue at passport control I ready myself for my first UK contact with officialdom. The

Border Control Officer is immediately unsure when I tell her where I have been working. She asks me to take a seat off to one side. I'm scrutinised by other passengers as they approach the desk. I feel guilty for no reason. I think I would be a pretty lousy drugs mule.

About ten minutes later a senior officer comes to talk to me. He says, "It's all fine Andy, I have called PHE (Public Health England) and they know all about you, welcome home and well done." He then shakes my hand. I guess I am generally quite sensitive at the moment as this act of kindness and rejection of fear brings a tear to my eye. I thank him for his time and kindness and pass through the arrivals gate.

Outside the airport I walk to the car park where Tracey and my Mum and Dad are waiting. After a brief joke about my being close to them we all hug before climbing into the car to head home. It is strange but nice to be back with them. It will take time to settle properly and I think we all know this.

# Tuesday, December 16

**Anna**
A lot of good news today. Janet, our staff member, is cured and has been discharged from the Freetown clinic. Everyone is very happy about that of course. Bindu, an 18-year old girl with an extremely high viral load when she came to us, a few weeks ago, is discharged cured this afternoon, very happy. Our little Musa is cured as well! I receive both Bindu and Musa on the outside as they are discharged, after my morning shift has ended. Such a great experience. In the counselling tent I give Musa a big hug. The boy remembers his aunt's phone number, and when the health promoters help him to call it, she is there and bursts out crying because she had thought Musa had died. So it seems he will be OK with relatives in Freetown. Shy and quiet Bindu will stay in the 'hotel' across the road from the EMC for a few days, until transport home can be arranged. Musa will have to stay at the orphanage, since he is under age. Sandra and I, with one of the health promoters, take Musa in a car to the orphanage, which has moved to a new location recently. The little baby boy with cerebral palsy, who miraculously survived his bout of Ebola, is still there and is looking very well; there is a young lady looking after him who clearly loves him, although I have a suspicion the women there are still hopeful that he may grow out of his condition. While there

we can also let 14-year old Mamani know that both her brothers, Abu and Alpha, are doing well. I am glad that we were proven wrong, and a kind of miracle happened: Abu has survived! He is doing better every day. I am no longer worried about him taking a downturn. He was tested today, and is extremely close to cure, so I expect the discharge of these two, our final confirmed Ebola patients, very soon.

Apart from Abu and Alpha, who are just sitting out their time, the EMC only houses one patient in the Suspect area (who is fine and will get his next negative test tomorrow, I'm sure), and one patient in Probable (who is ill with a lot of diarrhoea, but possibly not Ebola because his first test was negative). And that's it! Walking through the corridors between the tents in the High Risk zone is like walking through a ghost town. Until a week or two ago, these corridors and tents were full of patients, and you often had to step over patients lying everywhere. Now, the corridors are nearly empty, and several tents have been closed. While I walk through in PPE, I see the patients in my mind – in every tent, and in every spot in the High Risk zone, I have a memory of a special patient or a special situation. I see Peter again, the 30-year-old man worried for his sister but who died unexpectedly himself, though he had been a strong and healthy man. Or little Osman and his father. Poor Ishmael, suffering from convulsions, little Bobor or the young woman Sara, who miraculously woke up from her coma. Amie, who improved so much after speaking to her father on the phone, the boy Brima, our last Ebola victim, and three-year-old Tamba and his mother. Or the

12-year old boy looking after his two little brothers, who have all been discharged cured.

I'm the veteran expat working inside the EMC, now that Andy has left. I have to restrain myself from boring the other expats with stories about how everything was so very different four to five weeks ago. Or telling them the way of working when there were 70+ patients, that is now old news. The Kailahun EMC is being downscaled to a more 'normal' size with 20 beds (4 'suspect', 4 'probable' and 12 'confirmed' beds in 4 tents) instead of the original 96 beds – enough to be able to deal with any new incidental cases or suspected cases from the district.

There's more time to get to know the National Staff as well. One of the young men of the undressing team has taken to calling me his 'ma', for fun. He likes one of the women of the dressing team, and their friends have started to tease them about being a future man and wife. That would automatically make me the girl's future mother-in-law! It is clear that mother-in-law jokes are part of Sierra Leonean culture too.

Arriving home at the hotel at the end of the afternoon, there is a surprise for me. Someone is waiting for me, I'm told. Who should it be but the carpenter who promised Andy and me the walking sticks a couple of weeks ago! We hadn't heard anything from him since our meeting and I had almost given up on him. But he is here and he has brought two beautiful hand-crafted walking sticks, made out of one piece, both with individual details. He explains that the man carved at the top represents the paramount chief, the woman below is his wife. I forget to ask him what kind of wood he used, but the sticks are well varnished so I can decontaminate them with chlorine water without spoiling them. They are the envy of all the expats, and they make the local employees from Kailahun smile. The only challenge now will be to get them back home.

In my email inbox this evening I find a wonderful gift from back home. I had written to my colleague Chantal about Musa and his drawings and how he is recovering. Chantal's daughter Eva is of the same age as the boy, and was deeply moved by his story. So she mobilised her schoolteacher and her whole class of 7th graders and they have all made colourful drawings for him. I'll print them out and ask Sandra to get them to him. He will be thrilled with such an exciting gift, I'm sure.

# Thursday, December 18

**Anna**
After the morning shift, Elisa and I walk over to the graveyard to look for the graves of little Kadiatu, and Osman and his father. We find them in the far left corner. Osman's grave is near the edge. Unfortunately, his father is buried a little distance away. Kadiatu's grave is nearer. Next to Kadiatu's grave is that of Fatmata. I remember Fatmata. She was a 60-year-old woman, in the third bed on the left in C4. She was the grandmother of four girls who had all had Ebola and who were already in the convalescent tent while she was in C4. The four granddaughters were all cured but Fatmata died despite our efforts. It is nice to see that someone put up a more elaborate marker on her grave than the standard wooden stake. I like to imagine that the four girls arranged that before they left for their own district. I also like the idea that our two-year old Kadiatu lies next to her.

In the past few days I have grown more tired although our work is less intense. Or maybe it's because of this. It gives me time to realise all that we have done and seen in the past few weeks. My sleep is less restful than it has been; I wake up a few times every night, not because of conscious nightmares but just sudden wakefulness.

## Andy

From here I will add only a few days or events that were particularly meaningful. I am now in daily contact with the public health people who seem both efficient and very pleasant. They chat to me about the mission and about how I feel returning to the UK. I have all the phone numbers I need as well as clear guidance on the protocol should I feel unwell. I received a parcel today that contains the equipment they deem necessary for people returning from Ebola affected areas. This includes a tympanic (ear) thermometer and record sheet to keep track of readings, some chlorine powder, a scoop, some absorbent pads and some heavy-duty clinical waste bags. This is to clean up and decontaminate any body fluids should I become sick. Quite a scary thought.

For the first time in a month I am going to go running tonight. I didn't know what freedoms we would have in Sierra Leone so I didn't take my training kit with me. I set off about five o'clock in the evening, it is dark and there is a light drizzle in the air. I am going to run my usual course, which is about four and a half miles. It starts on a hill, which I am going to describe as massive. I am not giving any more detail for fear of being accused of gross exaggeration. I struggle to the top of the hill and cross the road. I am now on a long flat straight heading towards my old school. The houses round here are very posh and the Christmas decorations are in keeping with this. Once again my delicate mind is thrown back to Kailahun and to my last day in the EMC when I sat with Kadiatu. I can't run. I stop, as emotion overwhelms me, I cry freely and unashamedly by the roadside. After a couple of minutes I compose myself and carry on. I run into the centre of Harrogate and decide to call at Bean and Bud, my home from home coffee shop. As soon as I walk through the door my friend Hayden leaves the counter and comes over to me and gives me a hug. This sets me off again immediately.

Back home I reassure myself that this has to be normal after being in such a challenging environment. That said, I keep thinking about the staff and the general population in Kailahun. If I am this fragile after only one month how difficult must it be for them. I am hugely affected by this time yet I have cared only for strangers. They have seen and felt the loss of their loved ones directly.

# Friday, December 19

**Anna**

This morning, we find that Abu is ready for discharge. So around half past nine, both Abu and his brother Alpha go through the discharge protocol, take their final showers inside the High Risk, get a new set of clothes and are welcomed on the outside perimeter of the EMC by a large number of staff. Abu, who was probably a gangly tall guy before his illness, has lost a lot of weight in the last few weeks. His new trousers will only stay up when he holds them up, until someone finds a rope he can use as a belt. He has a nasty cough as well. We decide to treat him for possible secondary pneumonia and check him for tuberculosis. Ebola has left him in a weakened state.

The brothers join young Bindu, who is still waiting for transport home, in the 'hotel' across the road from the EMC. Their 14-year-old sister Mamani is brought over from the orphanage, and reunited with them.

That leaves exactly zero patients in the High Risk. No suspected Ebola, and no confirmed Ebola. Unbelievable. Five weeks ago, we were at 77 patients, with 10-15 new patients arriving every day. Since December 1, there has been a steady decrease in patient numbers. Today, which happens to be my last working day, we discharge the final patients. For now, that is. We are careful to impress on everyone the importance of keeping vigilant, of not crying victory too soon. Especially with Christmas around the corner. There is a ban on the celebration of the holiday in Sierra Leone this year; no gatherings of people allowed (except in churches or mosques). It doesn't take much to get a resurgence. The village little Brima came from still has 11 days of quarantine to go, since the boy was admitted with full-blown Ebola just ten days ago.

Nevertheless, the discharge of the last two patients for now, and the fact that the EMC is without patients at the moment, cannot go by unacknowledged. Someone has set up a stereo system in front of the warehouse across the road from the EMC. Loud happy music sounds across the whole centre, and many people dance: the National Staff and expats in the Low Risk, in their green scrubs and white boots, including the ladies from the laundry, and the undresser in front of the undressing tent; the carpenters in front of the carpentry workshop; the people arriving for their afternoon shift, in street clothes, along the road. Our last discharged patients, Alpha, Abu and Bindu, enjoy the scene as guests of honour from a seat by the side of the road.

This is my last day at work in Kailahun. After the two o'clock handover – with nothing to hand over – I decide to mark this occasion by walking back to the hotel with two colleagues. It is about an hour and a half's walk, partly through Kailahun town. A good way to say goodbye to Kailahun.

# Saturday, December 20

**Anna**

Today is my day for leaving Kailahun, planning to arrive at Amsterdam on Sunday evening. The UN helicopter will pick Jenn and me up from the local football field around one thirty in the afternoon. It will be my first helicopter flight ever, a new adventure to add to everything that has happened in the last few weeks. Not to put any further stress on my anxious mother I haven't told my family about it but let it be assumed that I will be travelling back the way I came, by car. Time enough to tell them when I get back home.

After a last lunch 'Kailahun-style', Jenn and I settle down in some chairs at the hotel for the final wait. Our bags are packed and stowed in the Land Cruiser that will take us to the field as soon as we hear the approach of the helicopter. Chatting aimlessly, we keep our ears strained to catch any helicopter sounds. But nothing.

At two thirty, Johan the logistics guy makes a call. Bad news: the helicopter flight has been cancelled and they forgot to tell the passengers. Apparently it has something to do with the UN Secretary General Ban Ki-moon who is visiting the region. So no flights today. For a moment, it seems an option to jump into the Land Cruiser and just drive all the way to Freetown to catch the plane leaving after midnight. But then reason takes over again: this would mean driving with hardly a break and through the evening, when darkness has set in. That's asking for trouble on the bad roads here, even if the police checkpoints would let us pass. We have to accept that we have just missed our chance to catch this flight. And the next one isn't until Monday night.

To be honest, I spend the next hour sulking in my room. It is such a disappointment, being all set to leave, looking forward to seeing my family again tomorrow and getting back to my own country and then it turns out that I'm stuck here. I'd timed the washing of my clothes so that I don't have anything really clean to wear now. After a while I cool down and begin to realise the pettiness of my response. The next flight is on Monday night, which means I will be home by Tuesday, just two days later than planned. We can spend the time with our friends in the familiar surroundings of Kailahun. I will survive two more days of the food here. Jenn has much more to lose, with her family in Australia, and now much less chance that she will be able to reach them by Christmas. I send my family a message that due to a hiccup in the travel plans I've missed the flight from Freetown and won't be arriving in Amsterdam tomorrow – keeping it vague like that means I can still avoid having to tell them about the planned helicopter ride.

Later, the afternoon shift returns from work at the EMC to find Jenn and me still hanging around. By this time I've accepted this as just two days of holiday in sunny Kailahun and can greet them cheerfully. It will indeed be a holiday, for the EMC is still empty of patients so they have no need of my services there.

# Tuesday, December 23

**Anna**
I arrive at Schiphol airport around five o'clock in the afternoon, about 34 hours after leaving our hotel at Kailahun. The trip has been very tiring but without any major events. There was no helicopter flight on the Monday, so we travelled back by car. At a brief stopover at the EMC in Bo, I met Alessandro again for a few minutes. He looked OK, having grown a beard in the last few weeks. As a logistics expert, he will be staying in Sierra Leone for a month longer.

A nice encounter at Freetown airport: the young man checking my temperature and checking the form I had to fill in with where I've been in Sierra Leone became very friendly when he found out I had been working with MSF in Kailahun. He thanked us for our hard work, congratulating us on the achievement of having no more patients for the time being, and wishing me a very good holiday, which I had deserved according to him – the news about the last Ebola patient leaving Kailahun EMC had already reached him.

Jenn and I split up at Casablanca airport this morning. She managed to book flights to travel on to Australia directly from there. If I'm grumbling a bit about the tiring journey, I just have to imagine Jenn's trip onwards to set everything in perspective. She still has more than a day of travelling to go but will be with her family on Christmas morning, Australian time, if all goes to plan.

My parents are at Schiphol airport to meet me. It is so good to see them again and give them a hug. We settle down at an airport cafe for a cup of tea and Dutch apple pie. My mother has brought the green cardigan, result of her knitting efforts. It's nice and warm, although a bit big. But that's not really surprising: I've lost about 5kg in the last five weeks and all my clothes are loose at the moment.

Before we start on the catching up on news, we have one important subject to settle. Yesterday, during my journey, I received a Whatsapp message from my brother Huib. It had clearly been difficult for him to write. It said that he and his wife Mireille had been thinking about it a long time, but did not feel comfortable with me being in contact with their small children before my 21 days of incubation time were up. Fear of Ebola. I'd been prepared for this kind of response during the MSF training, and had heard some examples from fellow expats. But I hadn't expected it in my own family. Huib and Mireille are very intelligent, well-educated and kind people. But it is as they said in training: this fear has nothing to do with intelligence. It is an irrational fear, like that of spiders, which can't be alleviated by the rational explanation that no spider you will find in Western Europe will harm you. If a rational explanation that I will do no harm to their children, that I won't bring them Ebola, does not help, there is nothing for it but to avoid them for a short time. We usually celebrate Christmas as a family, at my parents' home. Huib has offered to stay away with his children, so that I can spend Christmas with my parents. But of course that is out of the question for me: I won't keep the children from their grandparents at such a time. So it is settled: I will stay at home in Nijmegen and will skip Christmas this year. I'll visit my parents next week.

At seven in the evening, my parents drop me off at the hotel booked by MSF in Amsterdam. I fall asleep within half an hour and sleep for 12 hours.

# Wednesday, December 24

**Anna**

Debriefings at the MSF head office in Amsterdam, in a welcoming, good atmosphere, enhanced by the Christmas spirit. Everyone I meet at the office very explicitly takes care to shake my hand on meeting. That feels very odd: 'no touch!' is my first thought each time. I'm sure they do it on purpose.

When they hear about my changed plans for Christmas, they offer that I can stay in the MSF house in the small village at the Veluwe, if I want some company for the holidays. This house is available for international MSF expats returning from West Africa who for some reason or other are not able to return to their home country for the first 21 days, often because they do not live near enough to a good hospital to go to in case they fall ill. When this house was appointed for this purpose by MSF a few months ago, it made headlines in The Netherlands, with fear-mongers stirring up the village population with scary tales of Ebola being brought to their doorsteps. Luckily, things had settled down pretty quickly. I decline the offer. In my current mood, I don't feel like meeting new people and being sociable with strangers. In the afternoon, I take a train home. The last stretch between Arnhem and Nijmegen is in a very crowded train because of some train malfunction. Fortunately, I manage to get the last empty seat. It doesn't feel good to be in such a crowd. I never liked crowds of people before but this feeling seems intensified now. One thought makes me smile: what would happen if I announced that I have just returned from an EMC in Sierra Leone, working with Ebola, and this strange package I'm carrying contains two wooden walking-sticks carved by a Sierra Leonean carpenter from Kailahun? How quickly would everyone clear the carriage? I contain myself and don't perform the experiment.

My uncle and aunt, who live in Nijmegen as well, and have been looking after my apartment and post during my absence, pick me up from the station and drive me home. They are also so kind as to leave me to myself quickly after my arrival, as I just want to settle in back home again. They have been wonderful and have done fresh grocery shopping for me as a surprise, so I don't come home to an empty fridge. I find out that my brother has been to my house last week (which for him would be about two hours travel one way) to decorate the house with Christmas decorations and leave some gifts as a surprise, which is very kind.

# Thursday, December 25

**Anna**

A quiet day today. It starts off with measuring my temperature, which I'm supposed to do twice a day for the next 21 days. I keep a record, let's hope it will be a boring list of normal temperatures.

Some relatives call to wish me a merry Christmas. When they hear that I'm planning to go for a walk in the afternoon they ask me seriously: "Are you allowed to go outside, then?"

That walk is a good way to blow some cobwebs from my brain. I cross the river Waal by one bridge and back two bridges down, a 10km hike. When I reach the farthest point from my home, a sudden storm of rain and hail starts, so I get soaking wet and cold. It makes me smile to imagine that at that same moment it is about the hottest hour of the afternoon in Kailahun, and I would have emerged wet from sweat from the PPE if I was still there. On my walk I meet a lab technician whom I've worked with over the past years. She's actually surprised to see me; she had thought I would be in quarantine for three weeks at the Dutch MSF house in Veluwe. Another of these misconceptions! But she and her husband are nice, and actually do shake hands with me. Then, right in front of my house I meet my downstairs neighbour. I had not told my neighbours about the reason for my absence because I didn't want to make them nervous.

But now he asks me point-blank and I have no choice but to tell him the truth. To my relief he is fine about it and just interested in my experiences without any apparent fear. I have to watch getting a bit paranoid, automatically assuming that people will be scared of me.

**Andy**
Christmas day is very much a family affair for me. I manage to push Ebola and Sierra Leone to the back of my mind for most of the day and just enjoy the company of my family. I am enjoying being back with Tracey, though in truth we are taking time to get used to one another again. I think this is normal and in no way cause for concern.

My thoughts do drift to Kailahun just before lunch as the smell of my glorious vegan Christmas dinner wafts through to the lounge at my Mum and Dad's house. I think about the team still working in the district. They are mainly focused on outreach work now that the EMC is empty. It is vital to maintain the education and monitoring efforts in order to discourage or at least detect any resurgence of Ebola. I leave the lounge just for a few minutes and send an email message to them to say that they are very much in my thoughts and that I hope they can enjoy the day.

# Saturday, December 27

**Anna**
It snowed last night and is still snowing this morning. A white world outside although the temperature is still above zero. I have lunch with my aunt and uncle, the ones who looked after my house in my absence. A very friendly and low-key lunch but it did feel like my first real outing: dressed in nice fitting clothes, a necklace, hair washed, and actually with some make-up on again for the first time since Sierra Leone (not that I ever use much). Very different from the weeks in Kailahun, with baggy trousers and T-shirt, or sweat-soaked scrubs and boots, and hair just tied back. Back home a little before four in the afternoon, I get out the snow-shovel to shift some snow from the pavement in front of my apartment building. Not that there is a lot of snow but it is expected to drop to minus 6 degrees Celsius tonight, so tomorrow it will be frozen and much more difficult to remove. While outside, I meet another neighbour. It turns out he already knew where I had been in the past few weeks, through a mutual colleague, so no need for secrecy.

# Sunday, December 28

**Anna**
An unexpected experience this morning when I go out for an early morning walk. Half way down the street I realise it is not such a good idea. All the snow on the pavements and streets has frozen overnight and it is still freezing this morning. Even with hiking boots it is slippery on the icy bits and quite cold. I don't know exactly what it is but it triggers memories of the High Risk zone. I think perhaps it is the careful walking, making sure where you take your next step, which sets it off. I get tears in my eyes thinking about things that happened, patients that we cared for. It is masked from the few passers-by by the cold wind in my face, which can be my excuse for the tears. I decide to turn around early, and reach home again after only half an hour. I guess this is all part of dealing with what we've done and seen. I guess you need to go over it in your mind at some point to give it its place. I have confidence that it will be OK. Maybe it is just the suddenness of the memories that took me by surprise. Also perhaps the exhaustion. I have to confess that (except for the 12-hour night in the Amsterdam hotel directly after the journey) I haven't slept that well since my return. I still wake up frequently, without being aware that I'm dreaming or anything, and I don't really feel refreshed when I get up. I hope that it will just wear off in a few days or weeks. I write an email about it all to Andy.

Having been through the same thing together there is no need for much explanation with him and it is good to exchange our experiences. He returned home a week earlier than me so he can coach me through the first days back.

# Monday, December 29

**Andy**

This afternoon Tracey and I are going to Harrogate. We decided it would be nice to have a wander around the shops and to go for a quiet coffee. I have been back for two weeks now and things are slowly settling. I haven't socialised very much but my friends have been amazing. They make themselves available when I am feeling OK and take no offence when I say I need time alone or at least at home.

We arrive in Harrogate for about two o'clock and enjoy a drink at Bean and Bud before having a look around the shops, many of which have sales on at the moment.

About four o'clock we are in one of the big department stores when I notice that my legs have started to ache. I mention it to Tracey but really it was nothing. I feel totally well other than a vague ache in my knees. Tracey asks me, "Are you sure you are OK, there's nothing else is there?" I reassure her that it is likely due to my getting back into running and nothing to be concerned about or to report.

Half an hour later things have changed. I start to get a headache. It is very mild but I say to Tracey: "I had better go home, I think it's a bit more than just muscular aches." We set off immediately and 20 minutes later in Starbeck I say goodbye to Tracey with no kisses (which in itself indicates my increased level of alert). I walk to my house where I immediately take my temperature. 37.6 degrees Celsius damn it. The Public Health England rules are that a temperature above 37.5 should be reported. This is extremely low as it can be perfectly normal for someone to have a body temperature at this level and be entirely well. In reality I was going to call them anyway as I know that something is not right and we have to be careful to protect others and ourselves.

I call through to the York PHE office and tell them the story. I guess from that moment a series of events is triggered and I am inevitably going to be leaving my home in a very unusual and frightening way.

It is six thirty and I am sat in my spare room after a call from the infectious diseases consultant on call for Public Health England. I have a severe headache, joint pains (now all over, not just my knees), my temperature is 38.6 degrees Celsius and I feel light headed. I was dreading this happening. I am 99 per cent sure it is something I have picked up here and no cause for concern but I am awaiting an ambulance with crew in full PPE to take me to Leeds to the infectious diseases ward at St James Hospital. They are going to test me for Ebola along with an array of other diseases I suspect. I told the public health consultant about the two very minor PPE breaches mentioned earlier. I understand that they have to follow this through and I want to be as cooperative as possible.

Even though I feel confident that I have not got Ebola there is that nagging doubt, that little voice in the back of my mind that says 'what if, what if….'. In truth I am feeling a bit scared. I have told Tracey not to worry about me or about the risk of infection. I have not made physical contact with her since I became vaguely symptomatic with the knee aches.

It's eleven o'clock in the evening and I await the ambulance feeling both ill and worried, I am concerned for myself of course but also for Tracey and my Mum and Dad. I haven't told Mum and Dad about this yet as I want to know exactly what is going to happen before I frighten them to death. I email Anna to tell her of these events. We have been in regular contact since I left Kailahun and support each other in the transition back to normal life. I think she will appreciate the very abnormal situation I now face.

Despite my fears I laugh to myself when it occurs to me that I am maybe going to die anyway as Lorraine my boss will kill me if I am not in work on Monday next week!

I have asked Tracey to tell no one about my being unwell. This has caused a major problem at the public health office. A patient has just been diagnosed as positive in Glasgow tonight (a Save the Children returnee from Sierra Leone) and they are going to be extremely twitchy at the moment. Public awareness will be massively heightened by the events in Scotland and the last thing we need is panic. It is tricky to keep things quiet of course, whatever I do at this end, doctors and nurses will go home after their night shift and tell their partners about the nurse who is in for Ebola testing.

As I sit here feeling shivery and generally awful my mind goes back to those poor people travelling for six to eight hours in an ambulance to Kailahun from the west of Sierra Leone. I will be travelling in relative luxury and will be treated like the star of the show.

I took paracetamol at about eleven o'clock and steadily my temperature has come down. I feel a lot better at the moment. It's three o'clock in the morning now and I have just had a call from Jane the consultant in Infectious Diseases in Leeds to say that the ambulance is on its way, likely with a support vehicle, which will be parked 'around the corner at a discreet distance'.

# Tuesday, December 30

**Andy**

About ten past three in the morning I take a call from an ambulance officer called Stephen. He wants to talk to me about what is going to happen in about 15 minutes. Two ambulances (in case one breaks down) and two police cars (to keep the roads clear) have come from Leeds and are currently rallied at Morrison's supermarket car park about one minute away. To keep it as low key as possible a single ambulance will come to my house, I can then walk out to it where the crew in PPE will take me to Ward 20 at St James.

This goes incredibly smoothly: as planned, the vehicle pulls down my road and they shine a searchlight on to my house. I walk out of the door and to the ambulance. We set off immediately to meet the other vehicles at the car park nearby.

The two crewmen in the back are nice. One is going to Sierra Leone with UKMed (the UK Government's response team in West Africa) in February. One funny thing I notice is the ambulance stretcher. It has a cover on the top. It takes me a few minutes to realise that the cover is in fact a body bag! I say to the crewmen, "Cheers fellas, you know how to make a guy feel good."

As soon as we arrive at the car park the convoy sets off. I watch as the two police cars take it in turns to speed ahead and stop any traffic at roundabouts and junctions on the way to Leeds. It is very strange and it feels very uncomfortable that this is all for me.

We arrive at St James Hospital and I am given a facemask before being led past a few onlookers (staff) and to the lift up to the ward. I am taken straight to a side room where Jane the consultant and Ron a nurse both in full PPE welcome me. Jane takes a stack of blood from me. I also provide a urine sample and she does a basic examination. Ron tells me I am the first patient they had seen with possible Ebola. They are clearly new to PPE and enjoying the experience, which is totally understandable. When it comes time for them to leave they remove their PPE in a methodical and clearly prescribed way with someone shouting instructions at every stage.

It's five thirty now and I'm going to sleep for a while. Shift handover is in two hours, the day staff are in for a surprise when they hear about their new patient.

Eight o'clock and I snap into wakefulness as the intercom next to my bed chirps. Gale the sister in charge of the morning shift is calling to say hello and see how I am doing. She asks me to do my observations (pulse, temperature, oxygen levels, blood pressure), which I do, and my temperature is 37.5 degrees Celsius this morning. Everything else is fine. I still have a headache and feel a bit light headed so I take some of the Paracetamol that I was left last night.

At ten o'clock I call my mum and tell her about events. She is very calm and collected and just listens to my explanation. She seems fine though I know that she is worried. I reassure her that I am feeling a lot better and that it is just a case of being cautious. I vow to keep them informed of developments.

I receive a call from Jane about three o'clock, the bloods that were taken last night have been tested and are pretty much fine. Standard blood tests and malaria test all OK. However there was a delay in the courier picking up the blood, which has to be taken to the south of the country to a place called Porton Down for the Ebola test. It wasn't collected till half past eleven so it's likely to be midnight or later before the results are back.

I don't know what floor Ward 20 is on but it is high up. From my room I have a wonderful view of the cityscape and I gaze out of the window, lost in thought before going back to my chair where I sit and watch episodes of *Poirot* and update my journal. As the afternoon progresses my temperature creeps up again, it's 38 degrees Celsius by five o'clock and I can feel the joint aches and flushing starting to return. I buzz my intercom to ask for some more paracetamol.

**Anna**
Bad news from England: Andy sends an email that he has been admitted to hospital in strict isolation because of a fever. From his description it doesn't sound like Ebola, more likely a common cold virus. But it must be horrible for him and his family. I send him regular emails over the day, hopefully to provide him with some distraction in his isolated hospital room.

I spend the day with my parents. I decide not to tell them that Andy has developed a fever. No need to worry them unnecessarily. It's good to see them again. The sight of their front garden brings back some memories from Sierra Leone though: I had not realized before, but the plastic fencing that my father puts up around the pond when the grandchildren visit is the same orange fencing as is used at the EMC. This time it is a funny recall, I seem to be doing better today.

# Wednesday, December 31

**Andy**
At half past three in the morning my mobile rings and I jump up and answer it immediately. Hugh, a doctor I haven't spoken to before calls to let me know that the Ebola test is negative. I should be reviewed in the morning and if all remains well they will likely discharge me, reassured that it has been an innocuous bug picked up in England. Despite the ridiculous hour I text Tracey and my Mum to let them know the news (I was under orders to do so).

Early this morning Jane comes to see me dressed in just gown, mask and gloves to tell me, "Things are being de-escalated, we just need to check a few more bloods and do a throat swab and you should be able to go." These are taken and processed rapidly.[6]

**Anna**
Good news from England, Andy has tested negative. Of course, like I have been telling him and myself ever since I heard about it. But still it is nice to get the confirmation.

Despite that, I'm feeling more downhearted today. Standing in line at the bakery around the corner to buy the traditional fried treats for Dutch New Year's

---

[6] The tests later came back as a positive Mycoplasma infection, which in my case was a minor infection with no lasting harm.

Eve, there is a woman two places in front of me with a very cute two-year-old girl on her arm. Memories of our little girl Kadiatu flood over me. It's all I can do to just stay in the queue, buy what I want and reach home before I break down and cry.

Supermarkets are strange surroundings for me at the moment. All the abundance, luxury and choice. Such a stark contrast with the world of the people in Kailahun, who get their drinking water from the same river they wash their clothes in and who collect firewood for cooking from the forest. It's just luck that has caused me to be born here. All clichés, of course, but very acute for me at the moment.

A call from someone from MSF Amsterdam sets me thinking in a different vein again. "We are looking for help with the Ebola training in Amsterdam next week. Someone has had to cancel. Would you be able to do it?" I think about it for a bit, but decide to say yes. So less than two months after I did my first training with Ebola, in November, the new people going out will actually be learning from me. I remember, when I was in the training myself, how I was in awe of the people who had just returned from West Africa, who all seemed so assured. It will feel good to put my newly acquired expertise to use to teach the new recruits how to work safely inside an EMC.

**Andy**

By four o'clock in the afternoon I am cleared to leave the hospital. I pack my bag and head out of the room and through corridors I hadn't seen on the way in. I pass staff whose faces I see for the first time. It feels odd just walking away after all the fuss to get me here. No police escorts and no ambulances. I feel so uninteresting now. I leave St James Hospital and cross the road to the bus stop. From here I travel into Leeds centre and then to the train station. As I sit on the train I look around at all the people heading home or out on the town for New Year. If they knew what had happened two days ago, would they want to sit near me?

Arriving in Starbeck I walk five minutes to Tracey's house for our second reunion in two weeks. It is lovely to see her and we chat while she gets ready to walk with me to my Mum and Dad's house for a New Year celebration that I thought I was going to miss. This New Year will be a quiet affair with much to reflect upon. It is however wonderful to have a loving family with whom we can celebrate. We have so much to be grateful for and so much to lose.

# 1 year later

**Andy**
I have been back home for twelve months now but Kailahun has never left me. I think about the EMC, and the people I met there every day. This is partly because Anna and I decided to collaborate on the writing of this book. However, I cannot escape the fact that the month I spent in Kailahun was the single most intense period of emotions and camaraderie I have ever known.

I was and remain profoundly affected by what I saw in the EMC, the suffering and grief, the desperate and remarkable efforts of our staff to alleviate the pain and distress. We all felt the pain of loss and the joy of recovery.

My return to work has been difficult at times mainly due to my emotional fragility. At Harrogate District Hospital kind and caring colleagues surround me. My boss Lorraine met with me frequently in the first few weeks after my return. She wanted to check that I was coping with my return to work. There were tears then and there have been tears during the writing of this book.

My work with MSF continues, for now it is in the form of fundraising. I have a remarkable circle of friends who have rallied behind the cause of raising £100,000 for MSF. In 2011 I walked 2000 miles from Amsterdam to Barcelona to raise money and awareness. In 2016 Tracey and I will cycle 4000 miles across the USA from San Francisco to New York. My fundraising and other work for MSF can be found at www.andy4msf.com.

I have revisited Kailahun many times in the presentations I give as part of the fundraising work. I always talk about dear Kadiatu and how much her story affected us. When I show the slide of her grave marker it never fails to move me. Kadiatu and all of the victims of Ebola were not statistics they were real people who loved life and enjoyed the warmth of the sun and the cool of the evening. They loved and were loved. They matter.

**Anna**
The return to my regular daily job went pretty smoothly overall, looking back. My colleagues (especially Marcel) had covered for me in my absence.

Of course I was also still involved in the training for Ebola in Nijmegen. The safety procedures for dressing and undressing in PPE in Nijmegen are different from those in Kailahun. In February 2015, I was the doctor in a rehearsal with an ambulance arrival with a simulated patient. So there I was, in PPE, at the back of an ambulance, again waiting for the back doors to open to be able to look inside. That brought back many memories.

Even more so in early May 2015, when I was called at home, late on a Thursday evening, and asked to help out because a serious suspected case of Ebola had been announced and would arrive in our hospital in an hour or so. So I packed a bag with a change of underwear (knowing how I would feel after undressing from PPE) and jumped on my bicycle just before midnight.

It was a very different experience to that in Kailahun. I was in my own hospital and department, where I have been working since 1999 – no red soil or tents in sight. There were several doctors and a large group of nurses assigned to this one case. The patient was in a regular hospital bed. The Nijmegen PPE has a hood that covers the whole head and face, with an integrated air-filtration system, and a battery-run motor you hang around your waist, that makes a noise like a vacuum cleaner close to your ears. The undressing procedure in an enclosed decontamination sluice does not include the chlorine spraying that was such an integral part of the process in Kailahun.

But there were also plenty of similarities. The camaraderie among the medical staff, working as a team to care for the patient, was the same. The concentrated, careful way of working while in PPE felt very similar and despite the Dutch night temperature and the 'air-conditioned' PPE – the sweating after an hour inside was still significant, although less than at three o'clock in the afternoon in Kailahun. The feeling of relief when you undress is universal.

The patient did well. The next day we got the welcome news that he did not have Ebola, and the isolation procedures could be stopped. I went home early that Friday, very tired. After catching up with some sleep, I sat at home, my mind back on all we did in

Kailahun. I felt a return to the 'wobbly' emotional state of the first weeks after my return, caused by the flashbacks. However, this only lasted for the rest of the day – a sure sign of my overall recovery. And when I was involved in the care of two new suspected Ebola cases in June and July, I felt better about it.

Working on this book, together with Andy, has been a very good experience, revisiting our days in Kailahun, without shunning the painful things. On reflection it was an intense, and often dreadful time, which has had a big impact on my outlook on life. I have a better insight into the way of life in an African country, the impact of a deadly epidemic, and the wonderful work of MSF. We are so lucky in the Western world with our way of life and our access to everything, including good medical care.

 I am glad I went. Would I do it again if needed? Yes, without hesitation.

# Epilogue

**Kailahun**

Things are well in Kailahun, as far as Ebola is concerned. The boy Brima, who was admitted on December 10, 2014 and died a few days later, was the last Ebola case in the province to date. After we left, none of the new admissions to the EMC tested positive.

In February 2015, MSF equipped an isolation room in the city hospital in Kailahun. Local nurses were trained to look after any potential suspect Ebola patients. At the end of that month, the EMC in Kailahun was broken down.

One of the last tasks for MSF in Kailahun was the reconstruction of the large Ebola graveyard. More permanent grave markers were put up, as well as fencing and a tukul for visitors to protect them from sun or rain.

**Sierra Leone**

The country was declared free of Ebola in November 2015. However, a few new cases have emerged in January 2016. A number of agencies including MSF and the WHO continue to monitor the area since Ebola still smoulders in West Africa.

Since its identification in 1976 there have been nineteen outbreaks of Ebola. The 2014-2015 outbreak in West Africa was by far the largest. In this book we have steered clear of statistical or microbiological analysis of the outbreak. We have commented on the hope for new vaccines albeit with a slightly cynical viewpoint when it comes to the motivation behind their development.

We have told the human story, the story that matters the most. It is the story of the men, women and children that touched our lives as we tried to save theirs.

# Acknowledgements

The authors would like to thank the following people for their support, advice and patience:

*In the writing of this book*
   Anne and Mike Dennis
   Lorraine Dyson
   Tracey Hill
   Bill & Elaine Hulse
   Esmé Morrell
   Marian and Kees Simon
   Karen Thornton

*In our work in Sierra Leone*
   Our MSF colleagues in London and The Netherlands who gave us the chance to work for the people of Sierra Leone during this desperate time.
   The team in Kailahun both Expatriate and National Staff who inspired us and guided us during our time in the Ebola Management Centre.

This book is a personal project of the two authors, it was not commissioned or written by MSF.

# Glossary

**Analgesia**
Painkiller

**Cannula**
A needle-like device that is passed through the skin and into a vein. Fluids and medicine can then be given via this route.

**Cannulation**
The act of inserting a cannula.

**CFP**
Clinical Focal Point

**CHO**
Community Health Officer

**Confirmed area**
Area of the High Risk of the EMC where patients with confirmed Ebola are located. Tents are designated C1, C2 etc. within this area.

**Convalescent area**
Area of the High Risk of the EMC where Ebola patients are located who are recovering from their disease.

**Diazepam**
Medication for anxiety, also a muscle relaxant in convulsions

**EMC**
Ebola Management Centre

**High Risk**
Area of the EMC where patients are admitted

**Intravenous (IV)**
Fluid or medication given directly into the bloodstream.

**Land Cruiser**
Toyota Land Cruiser: Four wheel drive vehicle, standard transport on MSF missions.

**Logistician**
Genius fixer of everything from vehicles to computers, suppliers of medication and provider of electricity.

**Low Risk**
Staff area where administration and planning is done. PPE not required as no patient care takes place here.

**Med-Co**
Medical Coordinator. Based in the capital, is in charge of the medical aspects of the entire mission.

**Medical Manager**
Nurse in charge of the day-to-day overall running of the EMC.

**Medical Team Leader**
Expat nurse or doctor in charge of the medical functioning at project. Liaises with the Med-Co about specific clinical medical questions or problems.

**Mende**
One of the languages in Sierra Leone.

**Metoclopramide**
Medication for nausea.

**Mission**
1. The name given to an expats time working in an MSF project in the field. For example "This is my first mission with MSF". 2. The countrywide goal of MSF's presence. Each project is a part of the overall mission.

**Morphine**
Strong painkiller.

**MSF**
Médecins sans Frontières / Doctors without Borders.

**National Staff**
MSF employees from Sierra Leone.

**Nausea**
Feeling sick / wanting to vomit.

**ORS**
Oral Rehydration Salts. Used to replace the vital salts lost for example in vomiting and diarrhoea.

**Outreach Team**
Team going into the community for, among other things, health promotion, education and early detection of new cases.

**Probable area**
Inside the High risk area this is where patients are located who are strongly suspected of having Ebola (based on clinical judgement), but who are still waiting for the results of the blood test to confirm infection. Tents in this area are designated P1, P2 etc. See also Suspect and Confirmed area.

**Project Coordinator (PC)**
Project Coordinator – the senior MSF person in the project. Has overall responsibility for activities carried out.

**PHE**
Public Health England.

**PPE**
Personal Protective Equipment such as goggles, gloves, overall, wellington boots.

**Suspect area**
Inside the High risk area, this is where patients are admitted who are suspected of having Ebola because they fit the criteria. They are awaiting confirmation by blood samples. Tents are designated S1, S2 etc. See also Probable area and Confirmed area

**Triage**
Process of determining the priority of patients' treatments based on the severity of their condition. In this case, determining the likelihood of them having Ebola.

**Tukul**
A hut, usually mud brick walls with straw or metal sheet roof.

**WatSan**

Specialist in water and sanitation.

**WHO**

World Health Organisation